Honor Thy Symbionts

Jeff D Leach

ISBN-13: 978-1481258791

ISBN-10: 1481258796

The title *Honor Thy Symbionts* was borrowed from an article published in the *Proceedings of the National Academy of Sciences* by Jian Xu and Jeffrey I. Gordon in 2003.

Two organisms that combine and live together for mutual benefit are called symbiont.

Thank you for supporting the Human Food Project.
100% of the proceeds from this 'little' book go to support
our work in Africa.

CONTENTS

PREFACE

To paraphrase famed biologist Theodosius Dobzhansky, "nothing in nutrition and health makes sense except in the light of the gut microbiome." In *Honor Thy Symbionts*, the lens of our evolutionary past is focused on modern issues of obesity, GMO foods, diabetes, the rise in C-section births, ecology of our gut microbes, our African microbial origins, government dietary recommendations, probiotics *vs.* prebiotics, food poisoning, and more.

This collection of 21 short essays is not organized as a single book – with a beginning and obvious end. But a collection of musings ranging from 600 to 2,000 words in length. Though a wide range of topics is covered, a microbial thread connects all of the essays. This decidedly Darwinian (evolutionary) perspective is a nod to the reality that ninety-percent of the cells in the human body are not even human, but microbial. This makes humans super organisms – however, more microbe than mammal. This biological truth is reframing the scientific and philosophical conversation around *Who are we?* The ultimate questions of health and disease in our modern world will hinge on the speed at which we discover and accept that we have always lived in a microbial world and much that ails us is in fact discordance with the once symbiotic relationship we coevolved with these tiniest forms of life.

1

ARE YOU THERE AL GORE? IT'S ME, MICROBIOME

In the 50 years since the book *Silent Spring* sounded the alarm on humankind's poisoning of the biosphere with synthetic pesticides like DDT, the grass roots environmental movement has tackled issues ranging from clean air and water, animal rights and acid rain to the more recent mega issue of global warming. Despite these and many other efforts, a mere 19% of Americans report being active participants in the environmental movement, which might account for why humanity appears to be doubling down on its effort to degrade global ecosystems, putting us on a trajectory with an unfavorable outcome. But this might be about to change. Results of the Human Microbiome Project published this past summer may have unwittingly handed the environmental movement its Great Leap Forward by turning all of us into ecologists overnight.

No less than 200 scientists from more than 80 institutions published the results of the 5-year, $170M Human Microbiome Project in a series of major scientific papers. Though countless studies linking the trillions of microbes on and in our bodies to human health and wellbeing had appeared over the last decade, the results of the Human Microbiome Project has completely captured the public's imagination with all things microbial.

As it turns out, 90% of the cells in our body are microbial – making us more microbe than mammal – a superorganism, thus making the human body best viewed as an ecosystem. This biological reality and changing definition of *Self* is quickly making our current perspectives and views on nutrition antiquated. While we eagerly await the promise of that other genome project – the Human Genome Project – to deliver us from sickness and disease, microbiologists can predict with 90% accuracy whether someone is lean or obese from his or her gut bugs alone gut bugs alone.

While researchers are cautious and right not to oversell the microbiome (much work is still needed to confirm causation for many ailments), the direct or indirect implication of microbes in a staggering number of ailments and diseases of the modern world reinforces that we are on the cusp of a paradigm shift from the orthodox notions of health and disease.

While modern medicine will be quick to put into practice this new knowledge and accepting of its roots in the principles of ecology and evolutionary biology, the field of nutrition science, given its myriad and tangled history of stake holders and its entrenched notions, may be a little slower on the uptake. Nevertheless, the emergence of the microbiome as a key player in human health represents an extraordinary opportunity that cannot be missed.

Currently 50% of the world's population lives in urban settings, with that number set to increase dramatically as more people move from poverty to middle class. This reality has always been and will always be the greatest challenge to modern human health and to creating a global sustainability agenda for humanity. It is at this interface between the terra firma of our evolutionary past and the enhanced material standard of living that modern development promises, that ecological principles underpinning human-microbiome interactions and our success as species will allow an entire generation to reconnect with nature.

By reframing human health in social-ecological terms against the unprecedented shift from village to urban culture, we can move away from the tired rhetoric of "a calorie is a calorie" and "eat less, move more" messaging to a more thoughtful framework that recognizes health and disease on the basis of the ecological tenets of diversity, stability and resilience.

The shift to urban settings is characterized by improved hygiene and rapid adoption of highly processed westernized food. Though improved hygiene has many benefits, scrubbing soil from our bodies and food has thrown our immune system into an over reactive tailspin and is responsible for the skyrocketing increase in allergies and autoimmune disease. Researchers recently discovered that as the amount of glass and concrete in your neighborhood increases and the diversity of native plants decreases, the microbial composition of your skin changes and the risk for allergies goes up.

As we unwild our bodies, food and lifestyle, we reduce

diversity – changing the time-honored symbiosis of 'us and them' on which our immune system came to depend. For our personal health, rewinding our surroundings and being less phobic about dirt in our lives would go a long way towards increasing diversity and possibly have the knock-on effect of extending the knowledge of a diverse *Self* into a broader stewardship of estuaries, forests and agriculture.

Once we start down that road of awareness that the host-microbe relationship is an embedded part of the larger biosphere, we begin to start thinking about health as part of a social-ecological system and provide an on-ramp to connect the dots on the very abstract issue of global stewardship. The burning and clear-cutting of vast swaths of the world's rain forests begin to register as a moral imperative when considered from the very personal experience of the scorched-earth strategy of broad-spectrum antibiotics on your own inner ecosystem. In both cases, stability and resilience are tested – left untended; will either ecosystem return to its original or some altered state, with less resilience to future perturbations?

Just as invasive species move into recently slashed and burned ecosystems once bolstered by diversity, the clear-cutting bursts of antibiotics or slow eroding of resilience through repeated dosing opens the pathogens door to disease.

Further example of how ecosystems respond to perturbations is provided by the Deepwater Horizon oil spill in the Gulf of Mexico in 2010. The deep-sea oil plume caused a shift in the sea-going microbes, with an enrichment of species and genes capable of hydrocarbon degradation.

Our shift to an urbanized diet of highly processed and easily digested carbohydrates is somewhat analogous in that studies in animals and humans show a substantial shift in microbial communities when challenged with these substrates in their novel abundance. Since there is no precedent for such a diet in the evolutionary history of the human-microbe relationship, our westernized diet is best viewed as a perturbation. The impact on the long-term resilience of the microbial community, and thus the health of the host (us), is unknown. However, the precipitous rise in 'diseases of civilization' suggests we have shifted the equilibrium of our inner ecosystem to a new state.

Human-driven change to the global environment has many outcomes, of which climate change is the most prominent. Away from the public microphone, climate scientists have begun to think the Earth System is likely headed to an undesirable state unless dramatic and radical changes in governance and public behavior is experienced. It could be said that the health of humanity's inner-ecosystem due to urbanization is fast approaching the same tipping point – though our current disease burden suggests we may already be there.

Moral psychologists (yes, there is such a field) suggest that climate change does not register emotionally with most people in the same way that terrorist attack might, but if you could connect personal moral norms to climate change as a wrong that needs to be righted, then you stand a chance of rallying people to action in greater numbers. In other words, get people to feel it in their gut

So pick the 'meat issue' for example. If you think our

overconsumption of meat is contributing unnecessary green house gases to the atmosphere and contributing to global warming and squandering limited water resources, then connect it back to the human gut – a little closer to home. Researchers recently discovered that 42 known antibiotic resistant genes originating from antibiotic treated livestock have recently been found in the human gut microbiome and may be contributing to clinical antibiotic resistance in humans (proponents against GMO take note). This just might be the kind of gut feeling an entire generation of squiggly light bulb environmentalist needs to feel.

2

DO SPIDER MONKEYS HOLD THE KEY TO WHY WE GET FAT?

In early 2004, a team of researchers spent nearly five months in a lowland subtropical forest in Bolivia following spider monkeys – an arboreal primate that primarily dines on ripe fruit and leaves. From dawn to dusk, the researchers recorded every detail of the dietary habits of these wild spider monkeys. They monitored the length of each feeding event, categories of ripe vs. unripe fruit and young vs. old leaves, and so on. They took detailed notes on which parts of the fruits were preferred and collected samples of everything. Back in the lab, the protein, lipid (fat), starch, fiber and other micronutrient content of the 69 different plants eaten by our little primate friends were calculated. What the researchers discovered rocked the primate nutrition world and *should* create nutrition guidance ripples at the doorstep of every government or organization that issues dietary guidelines for its citizens.

In nutrition ecology – in which the rules apply to humans – researchers have put forth a number of models that govern why a primate would pursue a certain diet. It could range from 1) energy maximization (eat all you can when you can); 2) nitrogen (protein) maximization; 3) avoidance of certain toxic plants; 4) to limit fiber intake (too much bulk equals not enough macro- and micronutrients) and 5) nutrient balancing. Of these, researchers who study humans and nonhuman primates tend to focus on the models of *maximizing daily energy* intake while trying to maintain a *balance* at the same time. This two-pronged strategy is the basis of optimal foraging theory, which states that we must replace what calories we expend when acquiring new ones. Unless energy intake is counterbalanced with energy expenditure, then one's booty gets bigger.

Until 2004, primate researchers assumed fruit eaters were energy maximizers – that is, they would aim to maximize their daily energy intake. However, the detailed dietary studies in the Bolivian rainforest found that across all age groups and sexes, spider monkeys aim for a target amount of protein, regardless of how few or many calories from carbohydrates and fats they consumed in the process. In other words, the daily protein intake remained remarkably stable throughout the study period, but the overall calories from carbohydrates and fats fluctuated significantly. This meant the nutritional strategy was a daily protein target, *not* a balancing of macronutrients and a maximization of caloric intake. The potential implications of this study for understanding the modern obesity epidemic among humans are profound.

Amazingly, this "protein leverage hypothesis" – as it has been dubbed by Stephen Simpson and David Raubenheimer – is not confined to spider monkeys. It has been demonstrated in numerous other species including pigs, rodents, birds, fish and even insects. But what about humans? That answer came in a study published in 2011. Researchers from Australia and New Zealand measured the protein, overall energy intake and hunger levels in a 4-day study among 22 lean subjects. In short, the researchers found that diluting the dietary protein across meals with carbohydrates and fats promoted overconsumption. In other words, the test subjects would keep eating until they reached a target protein intake.

This would all be very academic if it weren't for the fact that overconsumption of energy-dense foods *may be* in large part to blame – along with rising rates of inflammation, shifts in the quality of carbohydrates, etc – for sky rocketing obesity in just about every corner of the planet. It's also interesting to note that according to the most recent *The National Health and Nutrition Examination Survey* conducted in the U.S., a drop in the percent of dietary protein across 1971 to 2006 was associated with an increase in total energy. Also note that stacks and stacks of peer-reviewed research has demonstrated that diets high(er) in protein are known to be more satiating and lead to longer and more sustained weight loss.

The findings among the spider monkeys has the potential for "understanding the evolutionary and ecological origins of human susceptibility to obesity." Since we share a common ancestor with spider monkeys, humans are likely predisposed to a protein target and in the case of our modern food supply of highly processed carbs and novel fats (e.g., concentrated vegetable oils), overconsumption to achieve protein levels is a highly plausible evolutionary mechanism contributing to obesity.

Since protein is the primary source of dietary nitrogen, which is needed for growth, why it's regulated and why targeted levels are required is seemingly straightforward. During our more preindustrial life, over consuming low-GI carbs and well-balanced fats from high protein but lean meats during the regulatory search for protein was not a problem. In other words, the "costs of eating either excesses or deficits of carbohydrates and fats on a given day to ensure ingesting the target amount of protein were small in relation to the costs of failing to meet the protein intake target." Furthermore, unlike unutilized fats and carbs, which can be stored and drawn upon when needed during periods of negative energy balance, no such buffer exists for protein. This suggests that the evolutionary drive to keep eating until a target level of protein is met is somewhat out of perceived control. (Note any one persons daily or weekly protein target will vary across gender, age, physical activity levels, muscle mass, pregnancy etc.)

Average protein consumption in the U.S. hovers around 15% of total energy consumed. The National Institute of Medicine — whose reports heavily influence the USDA's *Dietary Guidelines for Americans* — suggests a range of 10-35% for protein as a percentage of energy intake. At 15%, the average American is on the low end. Analysis of modern-day and historical hunter gatherer groups around the world suggest a protein intake on the upper limits of that suggested by the lab coats over at the National Institute of Medicine.

Endless studies of supermarket prices and the correlation with the energy density of foods consistently demonstrate that the best bang for your buck comes from highly processed carbohydrates, sugary foods and fats but not from protein (on average). Therefore, food prices – especially for those living on a tight budget – can create a bias towards less and less protein (that's unless you are down with eating beans every night).

It's tantalizing to consider how the relative costs of macronutrients (protein, fat, carbs) and our embedded protein regulation interact with the human desire for salt, sugars, our responses to display packages, busy lifestyles, built environments and so forth. A new field of study perhaps?

It is clear that environmental and economic change in our recent past has opened the door to obesity. However, we cannot divorce our strategies for dealing with obesity and associated disease from our biology. By combining biological and economic factors in our understanding of consumption patterns, we may improve health outcomes. However, current dietary guidelines and the backgrounds of the scientists and health officials who put them together seldom involve expertise in the biological and evolutionary realities of the population that they seek to inform. And this says nothing of the influence of the special interest groups that seek to nudge those guidelines in favorable directions. It's also sobering to consider that the very agency in the U.S. tasked with cobbling together dietary guidelines – for example, the United States Department of Agriculture – is actually an agency whose purpose is to, well, promote agriculture. Seems like a bit of a misalignment.

In our more distant past, access to protein and non-protein sources of energy was dictated by environmental constraints (deserts versus near-sea for example) and access to technologies (think nets, bows, spears) to acquire and process those foods. In other words, the playing field was leveled and humans lived in symbiosis with the landscape and its resources. Everyone had more or less equal access. Fast forward to today, and the costs of protein and non-protein energy is heavily influenced by ecological differences in the cost of producing those foods, issues of shelf life, costs of refrigeration and transport, and so on. Your economic status then dictates your access to this new nutritional landscape. Unless we figure out ways to produce protein from animal sources in a more economical way – that also reduces the devastating environment affects of animal production in the process – and promote the consumption of plant-based protein sources, we are unlikely to curb the obesity epidemic in a meaningful way. This all assumes, of course, that the protein leverage theory plays any role in all of this. Maybe it doesn't.

It may be time governments to shift farm policy and handouts to those farmers delivering animal and plant-based protein sources. If the costs of protein were subsidized – and the environmental impact could be dealt with – then we might have a strategy. In the meantime, give a wink to the spider monkeys next time you are at the zoo.

3

GHOSTS OF OUR AFRICAN GUTS

Every person on earth has two genomes. The genome we inherit from mom and dad is the one with which we are most familiar, and more or less stuck with for life. Our second genome, the one we initially acquire from mom as we pass through the birth canal, is more dynamic and made up of the trillions of bacteria that live on and in our body. This biological fact makes humans superorganisms – part mammal, part microbe. In fact, the cells of our human-associated microbial communities outnumber our own cells 10 to 1, and at the gene level, it's a 100 to 1. We are more microbe than mammal.

Collectively known as our microbiome (our microbiota and their genes), the seeding of this second genome occurs as we pass through the microbial-rich birth canal. From mother to child, this vertical transmission marks a time-honored step in our mammalian-microbe co-evolution that dates well before our Mio-Pliocene ancestor Ardipithecus roamed Africa over 4 million years ago. The legacy of this ancient relationship is evident today in the effects our microbes exert on our innate and adaptive immune systems, energy metabolism and the very structure and function of the gut. The fact that humans are colonized by specific members of the microbial community, and nudge other members out, strongly points to the evolutionary conserved nature of the relationship and the likelihood that our microbial partners even selected for aspects of our hominin genome.

The biological reality that we are vessels to a vast microbial ecosystem is radically altering our basic understanding of medicine, nutrition, public health and the very scientific foundation of what makes us sick. With an explosion in molecular, DNA-based technologies, the microscopic worth of the microbiome is now being linked to diseases and conditions as diverse as IBD, autism, type 1 diabetes, asthma, cancer, obesity, celiac, heart disease, neurological disorders, metabolic syndrome, and the list goes on. The evolutionary and ecological forces that are thought to have shaped our microbiome are governed not only by host genetics, but are profoundly conditioned by diet and lifestyle.

In just a few thousand centuries, our kind has gone from nesting in trees, to making stone tools and digging roots, to kindling fires, to subduing flora and fauna, to erecting massive cities, and finally to downloading Angry Birds over 1 billion times (and counting). For most of this march to mammalian dominance, our superorganism adapted to a nutritional and cultural landscape that literally changed at a glacial pace. But more recently, rapid adoption of technology and need to feed a growing population a shelf-stable food supply, along with hyper-sanitized food and water, increasing rates of c-section births, formula in lieu of breast milk and antibiotics for every sniffle, we are now out of sync with the microbial world. Therefore, it may be more correct to say diseases of modern life represent discordance with the ancient microbial world from which we all came and in which our guts are still stuck.

By yoking microbial biodiversity of the microbiome to diet, lifestyle, and changing cultural norms to the diseases of the modern world, a new paradigm in medicine that places humans in an ecological perspective is emerging. The current reductionist's approach in medicine that has emphasized studying disease in isolation, only involving human physiology and human genome, will have to come to grips with the realization that a vast and complex ecological community of hundreds of bacterial species and their genes may be responsible for the aberration of interest. Causality it seems may be getting a lot more knowable.

From this ecological perspective, the potential loss of microbial diversity with one-quarter of the earth's mammalian species facing extinction and the reduction in biodiversity in floral communities that are running parallel highlights the impact of globalization not only on terrestrial and aquatic ecosystems, but also its staggering impact on our inner ecosystem. Rapid changes in diet and cultural practices in the very recent past are homogenizing our gut microbiome and tinkering with, or worse, erasing, some very important evolutionary histories with our microbes.

If our microbial communities are a sum total of the nutritional and environmental landscape upon which we evolved, and cultural practices and even family history matter as well, then our human microbial ecology should serve as the backdrop against all diet and lifestyle considerations in our modern world. This also requires that we think about Paleo Diet not for the last 2 million years, but from the more ancient perspective of the microbiome and its relationship to our evolved adaptive and innate immunity, intestinal environment (e.g., bio-chemical characteristics of mucosal surfaces), and gut morphology. A deeper view is needed.

The subjective start of the Stone Age (which if the data holds could stretch back 3.4 million years now), or the arbitrary endpoint of agriculture, may be of much less consequence on our dietary needs from the perspective of the microbiome.

As the avalanche in research connecting the gut microbiome to a never-ending list of ailments grows more persuasive by the day, what is it that our microbiome and our ancient gut are trying to tell us? For autoimmune diseases, our gut is likely seeing ghosts among the trillions of microbes in our nutrient-rich intestinal tract, jumping, twitching, and over-reacting to friend and foe that seem to duck in and out of the oozing milieu. Our lives and food supply have likely become too clean, and we may be missing some "Old Friends" who once trained our immune system.

For the low-grade inflammation associated with type 2 diabetes, heart disease, and obesity, our easily digested modern diet and decrease in diversity of foods (mainly plants) is literally starving our microbiome, reducing species diversity and richness (dysbiosis), and providing ecological niches for opportunistic organisms to take hold. This opening of the pathogens door coincides with an opening of the once tightly regulated pathways to our inner systems. Our guts now leak, and we are likely witnessing the effects system wide, all the way to the brain.

Research comparing the gut microbiome of humans and other animals using 16S ribosomal RNA gene sequences provide some interesting insight into the diet our microbiome might be most accustomed, tuned our immune system, and kept our gut from leaking. When the gut microbiome of herbivores (e.g., sheep, cow, giraffe, gorilla, horse, rhinoceros), omnivores (e.g., ring-tailed lemurs, baboon, humans, chimpanzee, bonobo, spider monkey), and carnivores (e.g., polar bear, dog, hyena, lion) are compared, human samples not surprisingly cluster more closely with other omnivores. Interestingly, when compared to other hominids, humans cluster more closely with the bonobo diet. While bonobos do eat a small amount of leaves and meat, they are true frugivores, with a diet dominated by, as the name implies, fruit. Therefore, from the perspective of the microbiome, humans may be considered frugivores, although specialized, eating seeds and meat depending on availability. Flexibility is fundamental.

Deeper shotgun prosequencing of the genes encoded by the trillions of bacteria in the gut across these same diverse mammals, reveal that the microbiome of carnivores are endowed with enzymes specialized to degrade proteins as an energy source, while the microbiomes of herbivores like sheep and gorillas are enriched with enzymes specialized to synthesize amino acid building blocks. Humans, in this case, are more like the gentle herbivores than the top-level carnivores to which we are often compared.

The microbial component of human evolution is important to understanding health and disease as we undergo rapid changes in socioeconomic status and the amassing of populations in urban settings with less and less connection to our shared, and symbiotic relationship with nature. The fact that we can't, despite billions spent on genome research, predict with any reasonable certainty what disease you might get from our human genome, but can with 90% accuracy tell if someone is obese or lean from the composition of their gut microbiome, should be a humbling departure from our anthropocentric worldview.

As we look back for guidance on how we should go forward, giving more thought to the complex and symbiotic interaction between us, and them, will provide a framework that will more accurately represent the human ecology of our past. By seeing us more connected to the microbial world, and as members of simple-gut fermenters, the technological novelties that punctuate our past become smoothed-over with an immunological memory and a gut barrier forged over deep time, evolutionary time.

4

SHOULD WE BE WORRIED THE JAPANESE ARE GENETICALLY MODIFIED ORGANISMS (GMO)?

It's hard to find a pantry or refrigerator anywhere that doesn't contain food that wasn't grown, formulated with or fed a GMO (genetically modified organism). And that freaks a lot people out.

In short, GMO is a laboratory process of taking genes from one species and inserting them into another in an attempt to obtain a desired trait or characteristic – or simply turning on or off existing genes. And yes, this is different than grafting trees or breeding animals that farmers have been doing for eons. The difference, of course, is farmers are not trying to cross a tomato with a chicken – but the lab coats have been pulling off similar genetic tricks for some time and with increasing frequency. And again, that freaks a lot of people out (no matter how cool a glow in the dark gold fish may be).

People who are concerned with genetically altered

"things" are most concerned about food – more specifically the seeds used to grow those foods. The vast majority of the soybean and a big chunk of the corn in the U.S. are grown with GMO seeds (seeds patented and sold by the easy-to-hate Monsanto folks). While eyebrows raise when the discussion turns to genetically altered animals, like in the case of pigs that have been tinkered with to better digest phosphorus and thus reduce environmental impact associated with pig poo, tinkering with good old wholesome grains, potatoes, papaya, squash, and tomatoes concern a great many more people and governments.

At issue is gene transfer. For example, since Atlantic salmon only feed during spring and summer, researchers modified the genetic makeup of the fish by adding a growth hormone regulating gene from *E. coli* plus some mouse DNA. The genetic gymnastics enables the fish to eat year-around and presto, a fish that grows and reaches market faster. The big question on everyone's mind is what would happen if one of these *Frankenfish* got loose and mated with a wild salmon. Would this in some way adversely affect wild salmon populations?

If "horizontal gene transfer" were to take place, between say a genetically modified plant like corn or our salmon, might the gene gone wild have an adverse affect on the person who consumes it? That is, will this novel genetic material worm its way into our own genetic material and do something unexpected? The honest truth is we don't know for sure, and therefore many think we must ban GMO crops and animals, whether modified themselves or fed modified crops, until we do know. The scientists on the

"*GMO is okay*" side of the fence, and it includes bus loads of researchers who don't work for seed companies, say that while horizontal gene transfer should be studied it is unlikely to be an issue as it's *probably* been very common throughout mammalian evolution (and for my family members from the South, mammalian means us too).

While turning genes off and on is common in genetic research, using genes from bacteria for certain outcomes is more relevant to GMO discussions. So when we talk about GMO foods, we are – for the most part – talking about genes that have been harvested from bacteria and inserted into the target microorganism (say corn seed) to achieve a preferred trait or outcome. With most GMO corn, the donor organism is a harmless soil bacterium (*Bacillus thuringiensis*) and a gene that produces a protein that is highly effective at killing caterpillars. Harvest that gene from the bacteria and splice it into corn seed DNA and bam, dead caterpillars and higher crop yields.

Since the issue surrounding the safety and efficacy of GMO is centered on bacteria – and whether or not we can uptake these novel genes into our own genome – an astonishing finding in Japan surrounding sushi consumption is worth considering.

Reporting in the journal *Nature*, researchers from France and Canada studying how ocean bacteria break down marine algae (seaweed) discovered that a certain strain of bacteria (*Zobellia galactanivorans*) produce special enzymes that break down carbohydrates in seaweed into packages the bacteria could utilize as an energy source. It seems that when humans started inhabiting the island of Japan some 40,000 years ago, they began ingesting this marine microbe on slivers of seaweed and in the process introduced the special carbohydrate-reducing enzymes to bacteria that lived in their own guts.

Interestingly, since none of the normal (commensal) bacteria in the ancestral Japanese gut bacteria contained the genes to produce the special enzymes needed to break down the seaweed – and thus release its nutrient value – bacteria in the Japanese gut simply borrowed genes from the marine bacteria hitch-hiking on each mouthful of seaweed. Since the Japanese, then and now, consume sushi wrapped in seaweed, the evolutionary pressure to keep the horizontal gene transfer going persisted.

When the researchers tested for the presence of this special enzyme in the gut microbiome (collective genomes of all the bacteria in the human gut) of 13 Japanese volunteers, it was present in every person. Astonishingly, the enzymes were also found in gut bugs of newborns that had obviously never eaten sushi. This suggests that bacteria containing these special genes were *transferred vertically* from mother to child during birth. When the researchers tested 18 volunteers living in the U.S., they could find no evidence for the special seaweed-eating genes.

The clear-cut horizontal gene transfer of seaweed-eating genes from marine bacteria to human gut bacteria is more or less what the "no GMO" proponents fear the most. In the case of the Japanese, whose ancient and modern diet include significant amounts of seaweed in soups, garnishments, and wrap for sushi, the gene transfer was facilitated and maintained by evolutionary forces. That is, the human gut microbiome with its trillions of inhabitants did not possess the genes to produce the special seaweed-degrading enzymes, so it simply borrowed them from marine bacteria – and then proceeded to pass them down through generations. In other words, there was a benefit to do so – in this case, maximizing calories from seaweed.

Equally important is the fact that western populations do not possess these genes within their gut microbiomes. Why? Even though westerners have eaten seaweed throughout history, it has not been important enough in western diet for the bacterial genes from the seaweed-eaters to take hold and persist. In other words, there was no benefit to the host. And for modern western populations, even less so given that the seaweed that is wrapped around most modern sushi has been heated, and therefore all the marine microbes terminated from the heat.

The horizontal gene transfer from marine bacteria to human microbiome was a first for science – but likely not the last. This example eloquently demonstrates the important role of the gut microbiome in our evolutionary success as a species and clearly demonstrates that gene transfer likely only takes hold if the host genome or microbiome perceives a benefit.

As we continue to scrub the microbes from our daily lives – through antibiotics, wet wipes, and hyper-sterilized, cooked, and cleaned food supply – what important gene transfer events are we wiping away?

5

ARE GOVERNMENT RECOMMENDATIONS FOR DAILY FIBER INTAKE TOO LOW? AN EVOLUTIONARY PERSPECTIVE

Modern humans are the latest in a diverse line of species within the genus Homo that evolved on a nutritional landscape very different from the one we find ourselves on today. During the ~ 2.5 million years since the first member of our genus made an appearance in the fossil record, humans subsisted on an extraordinary diversity of wild plants and animals from a dynamic environment that literally changed at a glacial pace. It is only within the last 5,000 to 10,000 years that our food supply has begun to include domesticated plants and animals. For more than 99% of human history, our genome and its nutritional and physiological parameters were selected during our non-domesticated foraging life-way conditioned, in no small way, by a diet that included large amounts of dietary fiber from a significant diversity of sources.

Even though this important reality underlies the basic

evolutionary biological principles of modern human nutrient requirements, it is all but missing from policy and research discussions on recommended intake of dietary fiber throughout the world. Even more startling, much of our discussion on the health benefits of fiber, at least in the U.S. and U.K., often refer to the mechanical actions of fiber (stool bulking, for example) and nearly ignores the critical role of dietary fiber as a nutrient base of sorts for the trillions of microbes living throughout the human gut.

It's safe to say that our current chronic low-intake of dietary fiber in the western world (~12 to 15g/d) – coupled with our overuse of antibiotics and the increase in multiple antibiotic resistance in pathogens – has started a large-scale genetic "re-engineering" experiment on the slowly evolved and critical symbiotic relationship between humans and our little evolutionary hitchhiking friends, with limited discussion of its outcome on public health.

As you read this, there are millions of tiny microbes swimming around in the fluid surrounding your eyeballs. But you can't see them. There are millions more under your fingernails, on your hands, arms, legs and just about every imaginable section of your fleshy real estate. There are millions more lining your moist nasal passage, many more maneuvering about your liver, heart, lungs, pancreas and trillions more have been living throughout your continuous gastrointestinal tract – from mouth to anus – from the moment you enter this world. But this is good news.

The bad news is as we fill our shopping carts and pantries with the latest neatly boxed and wrapped goodies of industry, we continue down a path that began some ten thousand years ago with the emergence of agriculture – an event that eventually, along with steel roller mills in the 1880s, farm subsidies in the 1970s, and the divergent interests of food sellers and public health, may be leading us on a path to one of the greatest unintended consequences in human history by tinkering with the health of our intestinal microbes. Current dietary advice would be well served by an appreciation that the average human is a complex super-organism, rather than a single individual with one genome.

The archaeological and ethnographic record serves as an interesting reminder of the magnitude of the shift in the diversity and quantity of fiber in human diet.

Along the shores of the Sea of Galilee in modern-day Israel, a remarkably well-preserved collection of plant remains recovered from the 23,000-year-old archaeological site of Ohalo II provides an extraordinary window into a broad-spectrum diet that yielded a collection of >90,000 plant remains representing small grass seeds, cereals (emmer wheat, barley), acorns, almonds, raspberries, grapes, wild fig, pistachios, and various other fruits and berries. Owing to excellent preservation, a stunning 142 different species of plants were identified, revealing the rich diversity of fiber sources that was consumed by the site inhabitants.

In Australia, Aborigines are known to have eaten some 300 different species of fruit, 150 varieties of roots and tubers, and a dizzying number of nuts, seeds, and vegetables. Recent analysis of over 800 of these plant foods suggest the fiber intake was estimated between 80 to 130 g/d – possibly more – depending on the contribution of plants to daily energy needs.

In semi-arid west Texas, a nearly continuous 10,000-year record of ancient foraging reveals a plant-based diet that conservatively provided between 100 to 250 g/d of dietary fiber. Analysis of hundreds of preserved human feces (coprolites) recovered throughout the 10,000-year archaeological sequence reveal that a significant diversity of plants were consumed.

While the diversity and quantity of fiber varied spatially and temporally in the past, our ancestors clearly evolved on a diet that included daily intake of fiber from a huge diversity of sources that far exceed those recorded among populations in recent intervention and prospective studies concerned with the role of fiber in human health. These modern studies invariably group people with fiber intakes hovering around 20 g/d as the "high fiber" group, when in reality these high fiber or upper quintile groups are in fact low from an evolutionary perspective. Therefore, from an evolutionary perspective we should not be surprised when analytical hair splitting of these minute amounts of fiber does not yield the desired protective role one might suspect going into the study.

The potential protective role of dietary fiber among these modern studies may further be complicated by the lack of diversity as much as the quantity. According to data compiled by the Economic Research Service, United States Department of Agriculture in 2007, 57% of all vegetables consumed by Americans are limited to five sources (potatoes, tomatoes, leafy greens, lettuce, and onions). Unfortunately, the most consumed vegetable in America, the potato, is often in the form of oil-soaked french fries or potato chips. For fruit, five sources (apples, bananas, grapes, strawberries, and oranges) account for 71% of the total intake. From an evolutionary perspective, this minimal diversity, even when coupled with the handful of whole grains and beans/legumes consumed, translates into a striking shortfall in the physical and chemical diversity of fiber once consumed by humans and subsequently utilized by the hundreds of bacterial species that inhabit the human gut. We have changed the rules of the game between "us and them" in such a way as to possibly disrupt the organic harmony that evolved in this symbiotic relationship to a nutritional tipping point.

The emergence of prebiotics as a "super fiber" of sorts is just one example of the importance of diversity of fiber in the human diet. The steady clip of scientific papers demonstrating the health benefits of prebiotics is fascinating as we are literally peaking under the evolutionary curtain of our nutritional past.

Unlike probiotics, which are live microbial organisms that are naturally present in the human body, prebiotics are literally food for probiotics. While many fibers claim to be prebiotics, true prebiotics selectively stimulate the growth of certain probiotics known to be beneficial to humans, such as bifidobacterium and lactobacillus, while not promoting the growth of less useful or even harmful strains, such as clostridium.

Even though prebiotic fibers are present in more than 30,000 edible plants throughout the world, American and European diets only include 1 to 3 g/d – sometimes a little more, sometimes a little less. When we look into the archaeological record, like the west Texas example discussed above, we see daily consumption (though variable seasonally) of 10, 15 and often more than 20 g/d from desert plants such as agave, prickly pear, sotol, wild onions and so forth. Dozens of peer-reviewed studies have shown that test subjects who consumed between 5 to 20 g/d of prebiotic fiber, mainly in the form of inulin and fructo-oligosaccharides derived from chicory roots, were able to stimulate the growth of "good" bacteria, and increase calcium absorption, blunt hunger, relieve symptoms of irritable bowel syndrome, reduce biomarkers of some cancers, reduce inflammation through various mechanisms, improve immunity, and fortify our natural defenses against many food-borne pathogens. And the list goes on.

It would be a mistake to look at the science and health benefits emerging from clinical benefits of prebiotics as a new discovery of some magic bullet. More correctly we are simply witnessing a rediscovery of the importance of the diversity of fiber in human diet and, specifically, the role these particular fibers play in the health and well being of gut bugs.

The exciting science behind prebiotics coupled with the underlying biological reality that humans are *still* designed to ferment a large and diverse quantity of fiber (~50 to 90 g/d, minimum), and that much of our health is tied to the maintenance of a healthy population of gut bacteria, should serve as a wake up call for new therapeutic approaches to health. We don't need yet another diet for us, but desperately need a diet for our entire superorganism – both us and them.

Even though humans evolved from nothing more than a run-of-the-mill large mammal on an open savannah of other large mammals, to something of a geological force in an evolutionary blink of an eye, we owe much of our current success as a species to these tiny microorganisms. They require little more than a safe place to live and a steady flow of the quantity and diversity of fiber that they and their microbial ancestors evolved on.

Continuing to ignore our shared nutritional past with our tiny friends and adhering to the very human-like notion that we are somehow separate from nature will only result in progression of many human diseases to levels that will require the medical community to seek new vernacular to describe the public health hardships that potentially lie ahead. Fiber anyone?

6

KIDS ARE MAMMALS, TIME WE STARTED TREATING THEM LIKE IT

A child born in the United States today has a one in three chance of entering this world through a surgical incision rather than a birth canal. A recent WHO report found c-section rates in private hospitals in Latin America and Asia could top 50 percent, with rates in China nearing "epidemic proportions." With rates rising by 53 percent between 1996 and 2007 in the U.S. alone, there has been a lot of finger pointing to causes that might explain the dramatic increase. Whether its from being too posh to push or doctors wanting to schedule deliveries between golf rounds, virtually nobody is addressing the global health ramifications of what can happen when a mammal skips the time-honored "seeding" of microbes when passed through the birth canal.

Upon natural delivery, a human fetus is passed through an ecosystem of microbes that immediately cover and begin to colonize the newborn. A baby is born with an immunological tolerance that allows for the acceptance of these microbes that will soon assist the newest member of our species in defending against a daily onslaught of challenges from the microbial-dominated biosphere it just entered. Importantly, the microbes handed from mother-to-child will play an important role in the physical and immunological development of the gut and set the tone for a more complex and stable adult microbial ecosystem to come.

However, studies of birthing method have clearly shown that a child born c-section acquires a less desirable bacterial population more similar to the mother's skin, which is very different from the pioneering colonizers acquired during a natural birth. This disconnect with nature, possibly among all others, is unmatched in human history in its extent and its potential consequences to human health.

Our initial microbial colonizers have much to do with who we are, or about to become. According to Finnish researchers, c-section babies are at greater risk of becoming obese later in life, a finding consistent with the study of 284 infants by Harvard researchers. In both studies, researchers speculate early inoculation of microbes at the center of the problem. Further studies reveal a link between birth method and rates of asthma. And there are many more studies that suggest the same.

But how we enter this world is just the beginning of what it means to pull away from nature. Dropping breast feeding rates are adding injury to our biological insult of c-sections. While anthropologists have shown us that modern humans evolved on exclusive breast milk for a year or more, and extended breast feeding for two or more years, the CDC reports that 50 percent of the children born in Louisiana today will never breast feed. And of the ones that do, only seven percent are still doing so at one year. Breast feeding matters as it contains not only a well known suite of nutrients needed by a growing baby, but indigestible oligosaccharides the newborn's gut microbes need to flourish and defend against infection. Something not contained in the majority of the baby formula being peddled by predatory tactics in the maternity wards of every U.S. hospital.

The average child in a developed country will receive 10-20 courses of antibiotics by his or her 18th birthday. While life-saving in some situations, researchers believe the over zealous use of antibiotics may be leading to an unprecedented rise in irritable bowel disease from a disruption in gut microbes that can often stay out of balance for years.

We are rearing entire generations on a medical system not well trained in the principals of evolutionary medicine. Not to mention a portion of the general public is still not completely comfortable with our evolutionary past. Our modern lives are out of sync with our ancient bodies and mammalian rituals, and while our overconfident anthropocentric worldview has allowed us incredible control of the modern world, it is doing so at the expense of our microbial defenses and sacrifice of healthy years in life.

We desperately need an integrated public health approach that understands that our cradle to coffin strategy must begin with a restoration of our ancestral microbial ecology. We need to reduce c-sections, or at least empower parents with the information they need to make an informed decision. We need to improve normalization of breastfeeding in public and work spaces, making mothers more comfortable or able to provide her little mammal what it needs. And we need to think harder about the consequences of the greatest experiment ever imposed on the human-microbe population: antibiotics.

The First Lady has inspired a nation with a few vegetables grown on the South Lawn. Maybe it's time a nursery was opened as well, so mothers working in the White House could tend to the microbial garden of their children. Doing so will only improve the health of a nation.

7

DID OUR ANCESTORS REALLY LIVE LONGER THAN US?

In an article in the journal *Public Health Nutrition*, British nutrition researcher Geoffrey Cannon restated the widespread affirmation that "Paleolithic people usually did not survive into what we call later middle age." His underlying point, which is widely shared among researchers and the public at-large, is that our ancestors did not live long enough to develop cancer, heart disease and other chronic illnesses. All of which forms the basis for the near universal belief that ancient hunter-gatherers (our ancestors) really were not healthier or fitter than us moderns, and therefore their ancient dietary practices have little relevance to modern health, well-being, and longevity.

On the initial point, Cannon is correct. The average life span of our ancestors was short, compared to that of modern humans in developed countries where one can expect to live into their 60s, 70s and possibly early 80s, on "average." Conversely, a Neanderthal living in ancient Europe was lucky to live past her teens, and if you lived to your mid-thirties you might have been considered old in some early civilizations. More recently, the average life expectancy in the United States in 1900 was 47.3 years. By 1935, that age had risen to 64 years, and today that number hovers somewhere north of 70 for both women and men (though women can expect to live a few years longer, on average).

The first problem with this line of thinking is that the "average life span" math is misleading and tells us very little about the health and longevity of an individual, but rather gives us an average age of death for a given group or population. For example, a couple that lived to the ages of 76 and 71, but had one child that died at birth and another at age two ([76+ 71 + 0 + 2] / 4), would produce an average life span of 37.25. Using this methodology it is easy to see how one would come to the conclusion that this group was not very healthy.

However, the precept that diet played a significant role in the abbreviated average life span of our ancestors is simply not true. There are few among us that believe our so-called "westernized diet" of highly processed grains and added sugars and novel fats are an optimal diet for anyone – past or present. Our soaring rates of obesity and an ever-growing list of acute and chronic diseases – occurring in alarming frequency among younger sections of the population – speak to the discordance.

It is useful to point out that our species reached our current anatomical and physiological standing nearly

200,000 years ago. That is, while components of what we discern as hallmarks of behaviorally modern human beings, such as language, art, trade networks, and advanced weapons, have only occurred within the last 50,000 years, the hardware has been in place much longer. While we may drive around in hybrid cars today, we do so in very ancient bodies and with a genome that was selected, for the most part, on a nutritional landscape very different than the one on which we find ourselves today.

Before the advent and widespread adoption of agriculture, which depending on where you lived occurred between 1,000 and 9,000 years ago (or never in some places), humans organized in highly mobile groups of dozens or a few hundred individuals. Archaeological data and analysis of burial populations reveal that life was harsh and "dominated by warfare, strife, destruction, human trophy taking, and the all-to-often practice of infanticide." All of these facts of ancient life, in conjunction with the lack of simple antibiotics and modern surgical practices, resulted in shorter average life spans than many of us enjoy today. As agriculture took hold around the globe and groups settled down and built more permanent communities and ultimately socio-politically complex civilizations, the more homogenous and centralized food and water supply was easily contaminated by human waste. While war and even larger massacres continued throughout the agricultural revolution, tiny microbial killers took their share of victims, especially among the young and undernourished, further reducing the cyclical nature of the average life span. As European ships set sail just a few centuries ago, "new ills and evils further reduced the average life span of populations they encountered – albeit punctuated."

As war, contaminated water, killer microbes, and illness pulsed through humanity over time, our basic underlying physiological and nutritional parameters have changed little in the last few hundred thousand years. Our modern genome is in fact an ancient one and natural and cultural selection has built it to last. Under optimal nutritional conditions, such as those on which our genome evolved, we modern hunter-gatherers can live healthy and long lives.

We need only look to the modern Hunza of northern Pakistan or the southernmost Japanese state of Okinawa to witness the longevity that our ancient genome is selected for. With the threat of war and violence greatly reduced, and upon a sound footing of a safe food supply, our ancient bodies can be healthy well beyond "our best-before date" according to Cannon. Based on a low-calorie, high-fiber plant-based diet, a significant portion of the population enjoys healthy and active lives into their 80s, 90s, and often beyond 100. Incredibly, the aged portions of these populations have lower rates of obesity, heart disease, diabetes, hypertension, high cholesterol, cancer, and other chronic diseases compared to western populations.

The modern world owes much to antibiotics and advanced surgical procedures of the last half-century, resulting in dramatic increases in average life span for much of the developed and developing world. Though horrific events in Darfur and other African regions remind us how significant gains in average life span can easily be erased. In Iraq, a male or female could expect to live to an average age of 66.5 in 1990, but today following years of foreign occupation and endless violence, life expectancy has dropped to a mere 59 for both sexes – and slightly younger for males.

The self-confidence that comforts us today as we review the average life span of our ancestors is misguided and tenuous when viewed through the captivating haze of modern medicine that literally props most of us up into our golden years. I doubt our ancestors would call this living. While we may live longer than our ancestors, we are in fact dying slower. So rather than rest on our perceived cultural and medical success as it pertains to our longevity, we should challenge ourselves and our genomes to maximize our health for optimal longevity. For those not trusting of the past and the nutritional landscape upon which we evolved, our genetic cousins, the Hunza and Okinawans, have shown us a way forward.

8

STRENGTHENING YOUR BONES, NATURALLY

Osteoporosis. Just saying the word makes my bones ache.

If you're a woman over the age of 50, you have about 40% chance of suffering from an osteoporotic fracture. That's higher than your risk of contracting breast and ovarian cancer. Even worse, 50% of the osteoporotic hip-fracture patients never fully regain independence and more than 20% will die within 6 months. Not good odds.

If you are someone who thinks osteoporosis is a "women's disease," think again. It affects 25% of men over the age of 50 and an alarming number of young people. If the current trends continue, the problem is expected to worsen by 60% in the next 20 years – regardless of gender.

Most folks are aware that osteoporosis is characterized by bone fragility and related to dietary intake of calcium, or the lack thereof. Simply put – calcium is used to build bones and to a lesser extent, teeth. From the time we are born until our mid twenties, our bones are continually growing and require calcium to do so. The goal during this critical growth period is to achieve peak bone mass. Thick, mineral dense, bones. Your peak bone mass – which again, you can only control until your mid twenties – will strongly influence your risk of osteoporosis later in life. From our mid twenties to about age 50, the density of our bones is relatively stable. This means no matter how much calcium you consume, your bones are not going to get any denser. The goal now is to maintain the bone mass you developed in youth and minimize bone loss associated with aging.

This is especially important for women, who must contend with a number of bone loss issues exaggerated during and after menopause – not to mention the demands of pregnancy and lactation on bone health. While you are older and wiser, the efficiency at which your body absorbs calcium in later years, like so many things associated with aging, isn't what it used to be. Despite the fact that we are confronted daily with the "eat more calcium" message for "healthy bones" on TV, in newspapers and magazines, on annoying billboards, and along the aisles of our favorite grocery store, nearly 70% of Americans consume less than the daily recommended allowance of 1,000 – 1,200 mg of calcium a day – give or take. Our daily intake may in fact be lower when you consider that, depending on our particular genetic makeup and the composition of a given meal, our bodies may only absorb 30-35% of the total calcium advertised for a given serving.

Think about that little piece of critical information for a minute. Calcium that is not absorbed is mostly excreted in our urine and feces, which brings up an important issue –

and the point of why I am writing about osteoporosis – bioavailability. The terms "bioavailability" and "absorption" are critical nutritional terms that are often used incorrectly. Absorption describes the process of transport of a mineral-like calcium from your intestine across the intestinal mucosa (the wall) into the circulatory system, so that it may be utilized or stored by the body. On the other hand, the bioavailability of a mineral like calcium means the "proportion" that is actually absorbed and thus utilized or stored.

The key here is solubility. A swallowed penny, for example, has zero bioavailability. It will simply enter one end and come out the other, intact. Whereas a glass of water is highly soluble and will be easily absorbed – nearly 100% bioavailability. Even though you think you are getting 500 to 1,000 mg of calcium from a given food item, meal, or "supplement," you may not. Given this piece of information, it's not only important that we increase our daily intake of calcium to recommended levels, we should also seek out means to increase the bioavailability of the calcium that we do consume so that it's not wasted, so to speak.

One way of doing this is to lower the pH of your gastrointestinal system by delivering food to the trillions of tiny bacteria that live in your colon (specifically lactic acid bacteria). And that means fiber. Once in the colon, fiber is broken down by resident bacteria through hydrolysis and fermentation, which produces, among other things, short chain fatty acids and lactic acid. These acids then in turn make the colon more acidic, which increases the solubility of the calcium, making it more absorbable. One of the short chain fatty acids produced (butyrate) has been shown to induce cell growth in the colon, which in turn increases the "absorptive surface" of the colon. This means more calcium is absorbed and less is excreted in feces. Among the hundreds of species of bacteria living in your colon, you want to increase the number of the bifidobacteria and lactobacillus, specifically.

These two particular groups are known to be especially useful in increasing the acidity of your colon – and they thrive well on special inulin and oligofructose-type fibers that occur naturally in onions, garlic, artichokes, asparagus, and in lesser amounts in wheat-based products (resistant starch is great energy source for the bacterial community as well). They are also commercially extracted from chicory roots (think chicory coffee) and added as a food ingredient in a growing number of foods. These special fibers are known as prebiotics.

By increasing the bioavailability of the calcium that we do consume through a more acidic colon, we can add an additional dietary measure to the preventive strategies for fighting this terrible disease.

9

PROBIOTICS OR PREBIOTICS: WHICH WOULD DARWIN CHOOSE?

"Darwin" you are probably wondering, "what does he have to do with this?" A better choice might have been the Nobel prize-winning Russian zoologist Elie Metchnikoff (though few would recognize his name). He, like Darwin, exerted almost clairvoyant-like insight into biology and medicine, and his observation that many Bulgarians who consumed foods fermented with Lactobacilli bacteria lived, on average, to 90 years of age, effectively minted him as "The Father of Probiotics".

As for Darwin, a boat named after a dog and some swimming lizards on the Galapagos Islands is usually what comes to mind. And a pesky little book he wrote 150 years ago that people in Kansas couldn't seem to get comfortable with. None of which on the surface appear to have anything to do with probiotics and prebiotics. However, Darwin's wide-ranging worldview, experiments, and writings embraced the diverse disciplines of natural history, ecology, ethology, anthropology, genetics, and of course, evolution, making his potential take on it all interesting.

Metchnikoff was only fourteen years of age when Darwin made his big splash with his tome on evolution in 1859. By the early 1900s his bioprospecting in Bulgaria was driving the rise of a modern yogurt industry on the proposition that Bacillus bulgaricus, now called Lactobacillus bulgaricus, could transform the "toxic flora of the large intestine into a host friendly colony of B. bulgaricus." Like Darwin, and armed with the advantages of Darwin's wide-reaching theories, Metchnikoff's writings were as equally multi-disciplinary covering embryogenesis, pathology, and most importantly, inflammation and immunity.

But I like to think, if the advantages and transfer of knowledge were reversed, and it was Darwin who was armed with in some kind of crystal-ball-time-machine-thingy that provided him access to early twentieth-century knowledge of a practical scientist and pondering philosopher such as Metchnikoff, could he have made more of the tiny microbes and their implications for human health? Would Darwin have eagerly pursued and promoted probiotics as Metchnikoff had, or would he have thought more of prebiotics? (In order for Darwin to have considered prebiotics, he would have to set his time machine dial a little farther ahead, to 1995, when the concept was first introduced. But you get the idea. Keep reading.

According the World Health Organization, probiotics are live microorganisms which when administered in adequate amount confer a health benefit on the host. As for prebiotics, these are a *selectively* fermented ingredient (fiber) that results in *specific* changes in the composition and/or activity of the gastrointestinal microbiota, thus conferring benefit(s) upon host health. In other words, probiotics are live microbes and prebiotics are food for microbes.

Since probiotics have been on the research radar for nearly a century now, the published literature is massive, mostly paid for by industry, and not always conclusive. For prebiotics, having only been a concept since 1995, the literature is less extensive, but also mostly paid for by industry, and more often than not, more definitive.

The idea behind probiotics is fairly straightforward and aims to reinstate, more or less, balance in your intestinal flora and improve whatever aberration is bothering you. This runs the gambit from eczema, irritable bowel disease, mood and so on. Probiotics' weakness, in spite of overall positive results in some *dose specific* studies, is determining which micro-organisms are best and in which combination. The issue of dosage is also important and always complicated by degradation from things like manufacturing, shelf life and acidic human stomachs, all of which tend to reduce probiotic numbers before they can reach their target (the human colon more often than not). While "5 Billion Probiotic Cultures" on the label sounds great, those could fit on the tip of a pen. How many actually reach your colon where they might do some good? Manufacturers are working hard to address these issues, as a more discerning public gets wearier of claims on food and supplement packages.

From the perspective of someone like Darwin, he would

likely question the ability of a single strain of bacteria to impact on the vast inner ecosystem of the human gut. While we have recently only discovered that extraordinary diversity and richness of the human gut microbiome, Metchnikoff-era folks had some basic idea of the diversity of microbial life. A simple thought experiment Darwin may have undertaken may have been the analogy to a tropical rainforest, with its thousands of species of trees, flowering plants, mammals, birds, fish, reptiles, amphibians all encased in a warm and wet organic blanket topped with a canopy. The human gut is also warm and wet and home to tens of thousands of species and subspecies. Taking a probiotic – of any strain – and hoping it modifies your inner ecosystem in any meaningful way would be akin to planting a single species of flower on the forest floor at the base of a 200-foot tall tree and thinking this tiny contribution will tip the ecological balance. Maybe? But it would be fleeting at best and confined to a tiny plot of the forest floor.

This fleeting problem is what got the good folks over at DANONE in trouble with their commercials of Jamie Lee Curtis peddling the magic elixir Activia. Seems in order for the product to have any effect, it needed to be consumed multiple times a day, a tiny detail that Jamie forget to tell us. The $21M fine leveed by the FTC should help them remember to include that particular point from now on.

Darwin may also have thought that the concept of prebiotics was interesting, but may have asked, "why only stimulate the growth of a certain group of bacteria?" – similar to the rainforest analogy above. A nice body of literature clearly demonstrates that prebiotics, such as the special inulin and oligosaccharides (fiber) from chicory roots (the most commonly used prebiotic fiber), selectively promote the growth of bifidobacterium and other lactic acid bacteria, a group of bacteria that seem to be associated with reducing infection from pathogens, improved gut permeability, increased calcium absorption and so on. Importantly, a true prebiotic is selective, in that it does not promote the growth of less desirable bacteria like Clostridium.

As with probiotics, a certain daily dosage is necessary to achieve a bifidogenic affect, which appears to be around 4-8g a day. Unless you take a prebiotic supplement or fortified food – which the industry would like you to do – your best bet would be common foods like Jerusalem artichokes, dandelion greens, onion, garlic, leek, and asparagus. Although fibers with special prebiotic effects are found in more than 30,000 plants worldwide, most we can't find at our local grocery store (e.g., Yam Daisy) and the prebiotics occur in such small quantities as to be almost meaningless. If you are feeling enthusiastic, you could achieve a bifidogenic affect from peeling back and downing 1.5 to 2 pounds of bananas. A little less than 2 ounces of leek or garlic would do the trick as well.

From Darwin's ecological perspective on the world, he may have not advocated for either. His research into earthworms, which resulted in the publication in 1881 of his book The Formation of Vegetable Mould Through the Action of Worms, with Observations on Their Habits, which apparently sold as many copies as On the Origin of Species, may have also contributed to this conclusion as well. Unencumbered at his time in history by the free market machine of the modern world, he may have asked the obvious question of, "If the microbes of interest are already in you, why not just feed them and the other potentially beneficial microbes the diet they were likely selected upon over time, evolutionary time."

Working from Metchnikoff's observation that societies that consume fermented products seemed to live longer, Darwin may have reasoned that while bacteria in milk is interesting, maybe it's the totality of the natural environment of those milkers and fermenters – dirt, dung, cowshed and all – that support a time-honored symbiotic relationship with all microbes, not just the easily isolated Bacillus bulgaricus. His own well-documented ill health and homeopathic remedies, along with his observations of the symbiotic relationship between earthworms, soil and agriculture may have pushed him closer to our modern concepts of the *Hygiene Hypothesis* and *Germ Theory* for disease.

He may have also reasoned that as species change habitat and thus diet, they either adapt or die, but that evolution and adaptation take time, also leading to the observation that biodiversity in ecological systems result better functioning and stable communities. In the case of prebiotics, why just one, why not ingest a diversity of natural foods (fibers) that would promote diversity in the human-microbe ecosystem. This would broaden the definition of a bifidogenic or positive affect and free it from the bounds of regulatory or industry definition.

I suspect that the very nature of probiotics will change,

including who gets to sell them, what form they are delivered in and definitely the associated health claims. There is already regulatory rumbling, spurred on by the pharmaceutical industry, that probiotics should be regulated and held to the same clinical trial standards as other subsistence's (drugs) used to treat or attenuate disease. It is likely that probiotics will become cocktails of dozens if not hundreds of long-term community strains, delivered as a fecal transplant in capsule. Dubbed fecal microbiota transplantation, or fecal bacteriotherapy, the practice is showing some amazing results treating infections of the large bowel. So rather than plant a single daisy at the base of a 200 foot tree, plant entire fields seeded from the nursery of a healthy donor's intestinal tract. However, these precision probiotics of the future still do not address the basic problem of why a particular person is out of balance in the first place.

The same goes for the concept of prebiotics. A nifty concept that has drawn much needed attention to the ability to modulate ones intestinal flora with diet, it would be unfortunate if consumers didn't seize on this information and take the next logical step and improve overall intestinal balance by increasing the quantity and diversity of dietary fiber in their diet through whole foods. We will likely see more synbiotics as well – combinations of prebiotics and probiotics.

None of this suggest that yogurt with its billions of live cultures is a bad thing, or that a pizza crust fortified with prebiotic fiber should be avoided. With the avalanche of studies linking an imbalance in our gut microbiome to disease, and our ability to regulate this with diet and lifestyle in some positive ways well within our grasp, we are presented with our very own Bulgarian-moment circa 2013. The health of the planet is in free fall. If we don't start paying attention to some basics of human ecology, evolution, anthropology, and natural history, then we all might end up getting nominated for the Darwin Awards.

10

GUT CHECK

The ongoing outbreaks of *Salmonella* and *E. Coli* has drawn outcry from the media, predictable knee-jerk proposals from lawmakers, and understandable fear and confusion among consumers. As with past outbreaks, the Food and Drug Administration (FDA), Centers for Disease Control and Prevention (CDC), and food processing plants and farmers continue to take the blame for tainted food making us ill. But maybe our All-American sick gut deserves some blame as well.

While our attention is focused on farm-to-table food safety and disease surveillance, the biological question of *why* we got sick is all but ignored. And by asking why an individual's natural defenses failed, we insert personal responsibility into our national food safety strategy and draw attention to the much larger public health crisis, of which illness from food-borne pathogens is but a symptom: our sick, leaky guts.

The CDC warns, "The elderly, infants, and those with impaired immune systems are more likely to have a severe illness" associated with tainted food (and water). By "impaired" the CDC is saying that within the complex network of specialized cells and organs that work together to defend against attacks from foreign invaders such as Salmonella, something has gone wrong.

A critical component of a properly functioning immune system is a healthy, balanced population of bacteria. Bifidobacterium and lactobacillus, and other natural inhabitants of the human intestinal tract make it their evolutionary job to fight invaders by competing for nutrients (which the invader needs to survive), competing for attachment sites on our intestinal walls (which the invader must find to cause harm), producing organic acids (which the invader does not like), and changing the pH of the intestinal ecosystem (which the pathogen does not like either, but is quickly learning to adapt to).

This germ-on-germ warfare is fought daily. When the good guys lose, we know this as diarrhea, fever and abdominal cramps - or worse. And, while this germ warfare has raged in the human gut as long as humans have been around, the rules of war are changing as humanity has shifted to a highly processed diet that has altered the nutrient supply that friendly microbes depend on.

The irony of the public avoiding the fruits and vegetables suspected in an outbreak is that these foods contain dietary fiber essential to our gut bugs to fight the good fight. Our change in diet, coupled with uncontrolled use of antibiotics, may be adversely altering our organic relationship with our most important weapon against food-borne pathogens.

Increased gut infections are possibly having an

irreversible impact on our entire gastrointestinal system. Like a siege of cannon fire on the walls of a fortress, the barriers begin to crumble and allow invasion. Mounting evidence suggests acute and chronic infection by pathogens damage the delicate mucosal barrier that separates trillions of bacteria in our intestinal system from the sterile environment of our blood. As more battles are lost, the barrier and our immune system become impaired, resulting in inflammation and movement of pathogens (and endotoxins) into our sterile blood. An impaired and leaky gut plays a role in a range of maladies, such as irritable bowel disease, some cancers, sepsis, organ failure, heart disease, and a cascade of other metabolic disorders.

By inserting personal responsibility and some basics of host-pathogen germ warfare into the strategy for addressing food-borne threats, we may start to realize that we may not simply be experiencing a mathematical rise in food-borne illness as a result of sloppy farming and poor government oversight, but rather a tectonic shift in our nutritional landscape that has opened the pathogens' door just enough to glimpse the future of human suffering. Just the thought makes my gut ache.

11

FROM TURTLES TO TORTILLAS: THE EVOLUTION OF OUR LOW-GI DIET

Packed into four-wheel drive vehicles, ten middle-aged men and women traveled nearly two days on bumpy dirt roads and trails to reach a remote location, deep in the middle of nowhere. For seven weeks they would live off the land as hunter-gatherers, completely cut off from the niceties' of the modern world they were born into. Before embarking, each was weighed, measured from one end to the next, tests conducted, and blood and other samples collected. At the end of the seven weeks, lots of weight was lost and markers of major metabolic abnormalities attributed to diseases of their modern lifestyle were either greatly improved or completely normalized. They had begun to feel human again.

This wasn't an episode of *Survivor* or new twist on *Biggest Loser*. It took place over 30 years ago and those dirt roads stretched north out of Derby, in the northern Kimberly region of Western Australia, and the ten participants were full-blood diabetic Aborigines. In this relatively short reversal from urban life, the participants transitioned from breadavores and pastavores to true omnivores. They reverted back to the diet that selected the Paleolithic genome that they (we) all carry today. They had gone on a low-GI diet.

From Janet Jackson to Larry the Cable Guy, people everywhere are achieving and maintaining better health by paying attention to dietary strategies based on some basic and inescapable biological realities buried deep in our ancient genome. For 99.9% of the time that the genus *Homo* has been around (2.5M yrs), our carbohydrate intake was – on average – lower than the 250 to 400g per day consumed in modern diets (that translates into 1,000 to 1,600 calories a day). But more importantly than *quantity*, is the change in the *quality* of carbohydrates we are consuming today compared to our ancestors. And the glycemic index (GI) is a handy way to measure that *quality*.

"The GI is a ranking of carbohydrates on a scale from 0 to 100 according to the extent to which they raise blood sugar levels after eating. Foods with a high GI are those which are rapidly digested and absorbed and result in marked fluctuations in blood sugar levels. Low-GI foods, by virtue of their slow digestion and absorption, produce gradual rises in blood sugar and insulin levels, and have proven benefits for health. Low GI diets have been shown to improve both glucose and lipid levels in people with diabetes (type 1 and type 2). They have benefits for weight

control because they help control appetite and delay hunger. Low GI diets also reduce insulin levels and insulin resistance." (Glycemic Index Foundation)

Any farmer or rancher who raises chickens, goats, pigs, or cattle, will tell you if you want to fatten an animal before slaughter, just feed them high-GI foods (like corn) or feed laced with antibiotics.

For seven weeks, the overweight and diabetic Aborigines subsisted on a diet of turtles, kangaroo, birds, fish, crocodiles, figs, yabbies (look that one up!), yams, various vegetables, bush honey and so forth. In order of energy contribution at a macronutrient level, the diet was dominated by protein, followed by fat, then carbohydrate. Though they were "living off the land" and digging yams and walking around a lot, the researchers accompanying them were actually amazed at the low level of physical activity.

Contrast this diet with the urban setting before setting out on this little walk about. Back home the main dietary components were flour, sugar, rice, carbonated sugary drinks, booze, powdered milk, cheap fatty meats, potatoes, onions, and small amounts of fruits and veggies. Unlike the protein>fat>carb diet in the bush, the urban diet went carb>fat>protein. The latter should sound familiar, as carbohydrate intake in affluent countries average 50%. And thanks to decades of bad science and misinformation on the evils of fat, government recommendations on carbohydrates range as high as 65%.

Since our Aboriginal group was living a hunter-gatherer

existence, they did not have access to agricultural goods like wheat, corn, etc. This is exactly how all humans lived for the last 99.9% of human history (no agriculture). This meant that the carbohydrate (plants) we did consume – and that was consumed by our wayward travelers in the outback – was minimally processed. *Processing* can mean a lot of things that can range from the temperature and cooking methods (grilling, steaming) to the amount of mechanical processing (e.g., grinding, milling).

The minimally processed diet consumed in the outback meant that what carbohydrate that was eaten, was slowly digested and slowly absorbed into the blood stream and elicited a slow and limited insulin response (i.e., good quality carbs). Tests conducted before, during and after the 7 weeks in the outback, revealed marked improvement in how the individuals utilized and cleared glucose from the bloodstream and importantly, improved insulin sensitivity.

The improved insulin sensitivity is perhaps the most interesting result after the 7 weeks in the bush and the least understood evolutionary mechanism involved in how a low-GI works (note that *decreased* insulin sensitivity is associated with central obesity, abnormal cholesterol levels, high blood pressure – a cascade of problems known as the metabolic syndrome). As glucose is absorbed into the blood stream from consuming carbs, the pancreas excretes appropriate amounts of insulin, which in turn trigger organs and muscle to absorb the glucose. An insulin resistant person will not be able to absorb that glucose and insulin efficiently and thus it keeps circulating, unused, in the blood. And this is when the problems occur.

Though this may come as a shocker, the metabolic reality of our Paleolithic physiology is that we in no way need up to 65% of our energy to come from carbohydrates – as recommended by the USDA – not even close to that amount. Over the last 2.5M years humans have become steadily more carnivorous and what carbohydrate we did consume were *unusable* due to the large amount of fiber. It was not until very recently – circa 5-12,000 years ago – with the advent of agriculture, did humans consume energy dense and starchy foods with consistency. However, much of these energy dense cereals were coarsely ground or eaten in whole or cracked forms with large intact portions of fiber. These grains were slowly digested and slowly absorbed (i.e., low-GI). Our Paleolithic genome coped well with the high(er) carbohydrate but low-GI diet. But this was about to change.

The industrial revolution in the 17th century marked the era of the high-GI diet with the introduction of steel roller mills that produced finely ground flours with the fiber easily removed. These finely ground flours were easily gelatinized during cooking and thus increased their digestion and absorption. We in affect began mainlining glucose. And the rest is history.

Once our "modern" Aborigines returned their "ancient" genome to the low-carb and low-GI landscape on which it was selected, everything began to normalize. This low-GI reality means humans are innately insulin resistant. That is, a scarcity of usable carbohydrate, rather than food energy, and a high protein diet over the course of human evolution led to a positive selection of insulin resistance as a survival advantage. What glucose that was available in our ancient veins was used *thriftily* by our muscles and organs and redirected during pregnancy for fetal growth, resulting in greater survival of offspring. Hence why we are here today. So any diet that includes a significant amount of usable carbohydrates (e.g., pasta, white bread, sugary sodas), will only increase resistance of an already insulin resistant body. However, this does not mean that a heavy vegetarian diet reliant on large amounts and diversity of veggies will do the same – as a significant part of that diet would be unusable (high fiber).

Our modern diet has us awash in insulin and its myriad of metabolic problems ranging from weight gain, diabetes, blood pressure, heart disease, and more. Add to this the Angry Bird Era we have entered – at 750 million downloads and counting, it's estimated that 200,000 years have been collectively wasted by gamers on this game alone – our lifestyle has gave rise to an unprecedented body composition characterized by reduction in healthy years later in our life cycle. That is, disease comes earlier.

12

FARMER'S MARKET RX

OVER 7,000 strong and growing, community farmers' markets are being heralded as a panacea for what ails our sick nation. The smell of fresh, earthy goodness is the reason environmentalists approve of them, locavores can't live without them, and the first lady has hitched her vegetable cart crusade to them. As health-giving as those bundles of mouthwatering leafy greens and crates of plump tomatoes are, the greatest social contribution of the farmers' market may be its role as a delivery vehicle for putting dirt back into the American diet and in the process, reacquainting the human immune system with some "old friends."

Increasing evidence suggests that the alarming rise in allergic and autoimmune disorders during the past few decades is at least partly attributable to our lack of exposure to microorganisms that once covered our food and us. As nature's blanket, the potentially pathogenic and benign microorganisms associated with the dirt that once covered every aspect of our preindustrial day guaranteed a time-honored co-evolutionary process that established "normal" background levels and kept our bodies from overreacting to foreign bodies. This research suggests that reintroducing some of the organisms from the mud and water of our natural world would help avoid an overreaction of an otherwise healthy immune response that results in such chronic diseases as Type 1 diabetes, inflammatory bowel disease, multiple sclerosis and a host of allergic disorders.

In a world of hand sanitizer and wet wipes (not to mention double tall skinny soy vanilla lattes), we can scarcely imagine the preindustrial lifestyle that resulted in the daily intake of trillions of helpful organisms. For nearly all of human history, this began with maternal transmission of beneficial microbes during passage through the birth canal — mother to child. However, the alarming increase in the rate of Caesarean section births means a potential loss of microbiota from one generation to the next. And for most of us in the industrialized world, the microbial cleansing continues throughout life. Nature's dirt floor has been replaced by tile; our once soiled and sooted bodies and clothes are cleaned almost daily; our muddy water is filtered and treated; our rotting and fermenting food has been chilled; and the cowshed has been neatly tucked out of sight. While these improvements in hygiene and sanitation deserve applause, they have inadvertently given rise to a set of truly human-made disease.

While comforting to the germ-phobic public, the too-shiny produce and triple-washed and bagged leafy greens in our local grocery aisle are hardly recognized by our immune system as food. The immune system is essentially a sensory mechanism for recognizing microbial challenges from the environment. Just as your tongue and nose are used to sense suitability for consumption, your immune system has receptors for sampling the environment, rigorous mechanisms for dealing with friend or foe, and a memory. Your immune system even has the capacity to learn. For all of human history, this learning was driven by our near-continuous exposure from birth and throughout life to organisms as diverse as mycobacteria from soil and food; helminth, or worm parasites, from just about everywhere you turned; and daily recognition and challenges from our very own bacteria. Our ability to regulate our allergic and inflammatory responses to these co-evolved companions is further compromised by imbalances in the gut microbiota from overzealous use of antibiotics (especially in early childhood) and modern dietary choices.

The suggestion that we embrace some "old friends" does not immediately imply that we are inviting more food-borne illness — quite the contrary. Setting aside for the moment the fact that we have the safest food supply in human history, the Food and Drug Administration, the Centers for Disease Control and Prevention, and food processing plants and farmers continue to take the blame for the tainted food that makes us ill, while our own all-American sick gut may deserve some blame as well.

While the news media and litigators have our attention focused on farm-to-table food safety and disease surveillance, the biological question of why we got sick is all but ignored. And by asking why an individual's natural defenses failed, we insert personal responsibility into our national food safety strategy and draw attention to the much larger public health crisis, of which illness from food-borne pathogens is but a symptom of our minimally challenged and thus over-reactive immune system.

As humans have evolved, so, too, have our diseases. Autoimmune disease affects an estimated 50 million people in the U.S. alone at an annual cost of more than $100 billion. And the suffering and monetary costs are sure to grow. Maybe it's time we talk more about human ecology when we speak of the broader environmental and ecological concerns of the day. The destruction of our inner ecosystem surely deserves more attention as global populations run gut-first into the buzz saw of globalization and its microbial scrubbing diet. But more important, we should seriously consider making evolutionary biology a basic science for medicine, or making its core principles compulsory in secondary education. Currently they are not.

As we move deeper into a "postmodern" era of squeaky-clean food and hand sanitizers at every turn, we should probably hug our local farmers' markets a little tighter. They may represent our only connection with some "old friends" we cannot afford to ignore.

13

MICROBIOME SWAPPING, IT'S ALL THE RAGE

Parched, withered and feeling the burn is just another day in the life of a U.S. farmer this summer. The unprecedented heat wave pulsing across the Midwest Corn Belt is forecast to significantly reduce yields, impact a variety of other grains and seeds, and even raise prices in your local market for edible beasts. Though global warming enthusiasts are careful not to make too much of the current heat wave, it does add fodder to the debate and even more so for those who argue for more genetically modified crops (GMOs) able to withstand such droughts.

It's unclear if the general public will ever get comfortable with the idea of foods – plants and animals both – grown or reared from GMO seeds, feeds, and stock. The whole idea of gene transfer and tinkering with nature, not to mention the big multinationals that seem to control it all, just have people freaked out about Frankenfoods. But plant microbiologists might have a way around the problem – or at least until we decide their new idea is a problem as well.

Messing around with a grass (Dichanthelium

lanuginosum) that grows around geothermal hot springs at
Yellowstone National Park, researchers discovered that if
they sterilized the seeds before planting (that is, removed all
the associated fungi and bacteria), the grass would no longer
grow in the 160 degree Fahrenheit (~70 °C) environment.
In other words, there was something going on between the
plant and the bacteria and fungus inside and clinging to the
seeds that made it possible for this plant to live in such an
extreme environment.

That was 2002. Fast forward to 2008 and those same
researchers put two and two together and hypothesized that
if they took wheat seeds, which normally grow at 100
degrees Fahrenheit, sterilized them, and covered them in
bacteria and fungus harvested from the super weeds
growing near the geothermal springs, they would grow. Not
only did the spore-treated wheat grow at the scorching 160
degree Fahrenheit of the geothermal springs, it also required
50 percent less water than normal! They have also done
similar eco-gymnastics with other plants as well.

Now, you don't need to be a plant biologist, white-coat
lab technician or one of those farmers feeling the heat to
wrap your head around the ramifications of this insight. If
something as simple – well, not that simple – as swapping
seed microbiomes (all the microbes and their genes from the
seeds) could help crops weather the heat and do so with less
water, this might provide an alternative strategy to using
GMO seeds. At least those GMO variants concocted for
drought resistance (pest resistance is another matter all
together).

The microbiome swapping research among plants clearly

demonstrates that microbes play an important and symbiotic relationship with the plants. Although the exact mechanisms are still being sorted out, the researchers note that the plants cannot do it alone.

But the idea of swapping microbiomes among various plants – that is, the microbes and their genes – is essentially what folks concerned with GMO foods in general are, well, concerned about; gene transfer. Will this fact doom this creative and all-natural emerging subfield in crop science and agronomy? I hope not.

It's also interesting to note that throughout human evolution our ancestors' gut microbiomes were like huge gene vacuum cleaners, sucking up and sampling new gene pools as we moved from nesting in the trees to making a living on the ground. Perched high in the canopy, our earliest ancestors consumed the microbiomes associated only with the leaves, fruits, insects and other edibles who shared this aerial habitat. But as we began spending more and more time on the ground – and eventually figured out how to explore and exploit subsurface resources like tubers – we, I should say our gut microbiome – was exposed to a cornucopia of new bacteria and their genes. From this new metabolic network, it was not always necessary to acquire whole bacteria. Acquiring some of their genes was good enough as it's the genes, not the bacteria themselves that is what's most important after all. With these news genes, we acquired the ability to more efficiently degrade novel foods, such as the new starches and proteins that our gut microbiome did not encounter in more elevated previous addresses.

So as the range of our ancestors expanded with each new technology (digging sticks, weapons, fishing nets, clothes, etc.), we continued to experience new metabolic networks and borrowed from them what we needed. The evidence for gene journey is discernible today in the structural (taxonomic) and functional (genes) differences in the gut microbiome between modern humans and our close relatives, the chimpanzees (we share a common ancestor somewhere around 4-6 mya).

While we should demand to know what's in our food – i.e., GMO labeling should be mandatory – we should also bring all the biological, environmental, social, and evolutionary evidence to the table when discussing these important issues. Given the reality of our evolutionary past, modern humans are best characterized as high functioning zombies deftly controlled by thrifty, shape-shifting microbiomes. Seems our greatest fear may have already transpired.

14

SO GO THE PIMAS, SO GO
THE REST OF US

Anyone familiar with the American Southwest may have
heard of the Pima Indians of south-central Arizona. The
Pima are the modern descendants of the famous desert
Hohokam who occupied vast swaths of south-central
Arizona from roughly 200 BC to AD 1450. Famous among
archaeologists for their massive and intricate canal systems
built to deliver water to the arid and ecologically defiant
agricultural fields of the parched Southwest, the Hohokam
are a true success story of the ancient world.

While history paints the Hohokam as masters of their
ancient environment, medical researchers fear our modern
environmental landscape may be undermining their modern
Pima Indian descendants.

In the 1960s epidemiologists started noting an alarming
trend among the 11,000 or so Pima Indians living in the
Gila River Indian Community just east of Phoenix, Arizona.
For some unknown reason, a startling number of Pima were
developing type 2 diabetes.

Diabetes affects tens of millions of Americans, resulting

in the death of more than 300,000 people annually (and growing). It's also the leading cause of end stage kidney disease, adult blindness and amputation. The prevalence of diabetes among African Americans is nearly 70% higher than in Caucasians. Like obesity, diabetes dominates our national discussion on health care.

But for the Pima, type 2 diabetes and its complications are acutely devastating. With the prevalence of diabetes estimated at 5.1% of the global population, and more than 8% of the US population, the 38% recorded among the Pima of central Arizona gives them the distinction of being the most diabetes-prone group on the planet.

Once the trend started rearing its ugly head in the 1960s, researchers saw not only a looming health crisis among the modern Pima, but also an opportunity to study the disease in a genetically 'pure' group, as many of the Pima married within their own community. Importantly, they had multiple generations within families in which to follow the development of the disease and the genetic predisposition. With millions in funding from the National Institutes of Health (NIH) and the blessing and cooperation of the Pima, the Phoenix Epidemiology and Clinical Branch of the NIH was established.

It is now several decades and 100 million dollars later, and researchers are still grappling with the Pima diabetes enigma.

So why are the Pima prone to diabetes? Diabetes research in general has determined that lifestyle (diet, smoking, physical activity, etc) and genetic factors clearly play a role. For example, there seems to be a significant correlation between ones weight and predisposition to developing diabetes and suffering from its complications. But among the Pima, given the genetic isolation of the group, it seems genes may play a major causal role in individual susceptibility. Or does it? A new study may shed some light.

If you happen to be thumbing through a recent issue of the journal *Diabetes Care*, you would have come across a fascinating study by researchers who examined and compared adult Pima Indians of central Arizona with their genetic cousins, the Mexican Pima of northern Mexico. As mentioned above, the Pima of central Arizona are descended from the ancient Hohokam, who originally migrated to southern Arizona from what is today northern Mexico (several hundred kilometers to the south). Based on genetic, linguistic, and archaeological data, this migration is thought to have occurred a little over 2,000 yrs ago. Not all of the ancient population migrated and settled in southern Arizona, however, some stayed behind to farm the highlands of northern Mexico. This situation has provided a unique opportunity for researchers studying diabetes and other diseases among the Pima of southern Arizona. On the one hand, you have Pima who have embraced the modern western civilization and its lifestyle (diet) as it swept over them, and on the other, you have genetically identical 'cousins' who essentially stayed on the farm.

The Mexican Pima live in remote areas of the Sierra Madre Mountains and enjoy few modern amenities. Much of these communities only recently became accessible by road. The Mexican Pima are primarily farmers and work manual labor jobs, such as those available in local sawmills. Almost every aspect of daily life includes physical activity.

In contrast, the Pima of southern Arizona, who were traditionally farmers, "enjoy" a typical US lifestyle of computers and TVs, with low levels of occupational physical activity. They have ready access to automobiles and mechanized farm equipment for those who still farm. Indeed, two very different worlds.

The researchers set out to test the following question by examining adults among the genetically similar but environmentally different sets of Pima: "Do type 2 diabetes and obesity have genetic and environmental determinants?" In other words, does environment (diet, obesity, physical activity, and other risk factors) play a role in the development of diabetes when you hold the genetic pool relatively constant? If genetics played a major role in the southern Arizona Pima's astounding rate of type 2 diabetes, you would expect to see elevated levels in the Mexican Pima.

To add an additional variable to their study, the researchers also included Mexicans living in the same environment as the Mexican Pima in the Sierra Madre Mountains. The Mexicans (not of Pima heritage) are a mix of local Indians and Spanish. Like the Mexican Pima, the Mexicans live a rural and physically demanding life as farmers and ranchers.

Using Spanish-speaking interviewers and medical technicians, the data was collected. A brief medical history and physical activity questionnaire was completed on each participating individual, followed by measurements of blood pressure, and a 75-g oral glucose tolerance test. The entire sequence was performed on 193 adult male and female non-Pima Mexicans and 224 Mexican Pima near the town of Maycoba in the Sierra Madre Mountains of northern Mexico. In addition, obesity was assessed by BMI (weight in kg divided by the square of the height in meters), body fat was measured, and waist-to-hip ratio was determined. On top of all that, a 24-hour dietary recall was conducted to determine what everyone was eating.

Using the data collected from these two groups, researchers compared the obesity, diet and prevalence of diabetes to some 888 Pima from southern Arizona. The prevalence of diabetes among the three groups is presented graphically below.

The prevalence of diabetes between the two genetically similar Pima groups is striking. Among the Mexican Pima men, 5.6% had diabetes, along with 8.5% of the women. Compare this to the Pima Indians of Arizona where 34.2% of the men have diabetes and 40.8% of the women. Among the non-Pima Mexicans (no shared heritage with the Pima), 5% of the women were diabetic and none of the men. That last part is worth repeating: none of the non-Pima Mexican men had diabetes!

In other words, age- and sex-adjusted prevalence of diabetes in U.S. Pima Indians was 5.5 times higher than their Mexican cousins and 16 times higher than the non-Pima Mexicans. The researchers also point out that the differences seen between the two Mexican groups was not significantly different (i.e., basically the same).

The differences between the prevalence of diabetes

among the Pima Indians of Arizona versus the non-Pima Mexicans and Mexican Pima was also paralleled by differences in obesity, physical activity and diet.

BMI, percent body fat, waist and hip ratios were about the same between the two Mexican groups, but significantly different from the U.S. Pima Indians. The average non-Pima Mexican weighed in around 158 pounds (72 kg), with the average Mexican Pima at 145 pounds (66 kg). However, the average U.S Pima Indian male weighed 215 pounds (98 kg). While the women in all three groups weighed less, they followed much the same trend with U.S. Pima Indian females weighing, on average, about 200 pounds (91 kg).

As you may already sense, the levels of moderate to heavy physical activity among the groups was higher for the non-Mexican Pima and the Mexican Pima compared to the U.S. Pima Indians. For example, the average U.S. Pima Indian women spent 3.1 hours a week on moderate to demanding physical activity compared to 22 hours per week recorded for her Mexican Pima cousin.

As for diet, nothing glaring jumps out between the non-Mexican Pima and Mexican Pima – other than a remarkably low percentage of calories derived from fat, ~25%. In the current study, the researchers did not collect dietary data on the U.S. Pima Indians. Previous studies, however, reveal that percentage of calories from fat for U.S. Pima Indians was much higher than the 25% recorded for the Mexicans groups.

The dietary fiber measured in the diet among the non-Pima Mexicans and the Mexican Pimas deserves some special mention. No matter if they were male or female, non-Pima Mexican or Mexican Pima; they consumed greater than 50 grams of dietary fiber a day. Compare this to the 12 to 15 grams a day the average U.S. Pima Indian, or the average American for that matter, are consuming.

Given the similar genetic background between the U.S. Pima Indians and the Mexican Pima, the nearly fivefold increase in diabetes among the U.S. Pima can only be attributed to differences in lifestyle and environments.

While researchers continue to look for genes that make someone of a distinct genetic group susceptible to diabetes and other diseases such as heart disease, the current study among the westernized and nonwesternized Pima has taught us that obesity and physical activity have much to do with the likelihood that you will develop diabetes, regardless of your genetic makeup.

The take home message from the current study is profound: the genetic likelihood that you will develop type 2 diabetes is *not* inevitable and is *clearly preventable* if you balance a reasonable amount of energy intake with energy expenditure and follow a diet low in westernized, highly processed foods.

However, the escalated levels of diabetes among the U.S. Pima and the increase of prevalence with age (for example, 77% of the U.S. Pima > than 55 years of age have diabetes) hint at some underlying genetic discordance with the modern food supply and environment. This is what keeps millions of tax dollars flowing into the genetic-arm of modern medical studies among the U.S. Pima Indians of southern Arizona.

I would add to the current study that the dramatic shift

(drop) in dietary fiber in the U.S. Pima Indian diet from that of their Hohokam and earlier ancestors (who consistently consumed >100 grams of dietary fiber from a diverse variety of plants), has dramatically influenced the amount of insulin secreted throughout life contributing to the metabolic condition of insulin resistance – a complication associated with type 2 diabetes. This metabolic condition, which I call The Human Hybrid Theory, potentially affects all modern humans who have shifted away from a diversity and quantity of dietary fiber that our ancestors once enjoyed and that our genome was selected upon.

It is worth noting that the non-Pima Mexican men, a group that recorded the highest consumption of fiber at 56 grams a day, not a single case of diabetes was noted. Not one.

15

IF ONLY VEGETABLES SMELLED AS GOOD AS BACON

I often peruse the *Loss-Adjusted Food Availability* spreadsheets available on the USDA's Economic Research Service (ERS) website for updates (I know, get a life). Despite the boring title, the data is quite interesting as it provides per capita food availability in the U.S., adjusted for food spoilage, plate waste, "other" losses, and what we export and import. In short, what farmers grow minus what gets tossed before and after a meal equals what Americans are consuming, more or less, of various foods over time. Though the data are not perfect, and could even be consider too coarse-grained for most analysis, they do provide insight into some interesting trends. Economists at the USDA have been tracking this data in massive excel spreadsheets since 1970.

Even though this data does not measure actual consumption, that's done by the good folks over at the *National Health and Nutrition Examination Surveys*, and the data is alarming.

According to the economists at the ERS, the "average"

American (all age groups) consumed 2,594 calories in 2009. Of that, 619 (24%) of those calories came from flour and cereal products (wheat, rice corn, etc.), 596 (23%) from added fats, oil, and dairy fats (butter, margarine, lard, salad and cooking oils, half and half, etc), 473 (18%) from meat, eggs and nuts, 440 (17%) from caloric sweeteners and 261 (10%) from dairy products. Perhaps most striking is the so few calories in the average American diet that are derived from vegetables and fruit.

A mere 87 (3%) calories a day for fruits and 118 (5%) calories from vegetables. We all know that many fruits and veggies are predominately water, but 87 calories from fruits! Really? If my math is correct – and to put it into perspective – 87 calories of fruit is equivalent to 8-9 McDonald's French fries.

Of the veggies consumed, a whopping 47% were potatoes (e.g., chips, french fries). Other movers in the veggie category included carrots, onions, beans, legumes, cucumbers, and sweet corn – but all were in the single digits.

Despite the never-ending messaging to consume more fruits and veggies from every nutritional corner on earth, and the government's "eat 5 servings of fruits and vegetables" initiatives (think *5 A Day* program, which is now 5-9 servings a day), fruit and vegetable consumption has remained more or less flat over the past 40 years. However, we have seen a steady rise – and even some striking spikes – in other categories.

Interestingly, the government-sponsored *5 A Day* program, which was founded in 1991 by the National Cancer Institute and the National Institutes of Health, was farmed out a few years ago to the Produce for Better Health Foundation, which relies on support from private industry to get out their *Fruits & Veggies More Matters* message.

As calculated by the ERS researchers, the average daily calories from fruits and veggies above translate into 0.9 servings a day of fruit and 1.7 servings a day for vegetables, for a total of 2.6 servings a day. Even doubling that number to reach the minimum recommended 5 servings a day, something that has not been possible in nearly 40 years, would also mean doubling production. Doubling, much less tripling produce production in the U.S., is much harder than it sounds and likely means more imports – something that freaks out the food safety folks given the soaring land prices in the U.S. (i.e., all the good arable land is taken up with existing crops, cows or pavement).

This is why the launch of the USDA's new *MyPlate*, and Harvard's dueling *Healthy Eating Plate*, are not likely to get average Americans to consume more fruits and veggies. The messaging is the same, so the results will not be any better (history is our guide here). To honestly increase produce consumption to reasonable levels – what ever that is – will require significant policy initiatives/changes from the top down. We will need to go beyond a poorly funded *MyPlate* program and overhaul the system fencerow to fencerow and all the way to the grocery isle and classrooms of America. That means farm subsidies, looking at predatory marketing by food companies, addressing social inequalities from WIC to grocery stores in disadvantaged neighborhoods, better planned communities, and dare I say, teaching underlying biological principles of human evolution and genetics that are selected for our current nutritional needs.

Unfeigned biologically driven education + policy is what will move the needle.

16

GUTS, GERMS AND MEALS: WHAT 37 MICROBIOLOGIST SAY ABOUT DIET

Early in 2011, U.S. News & World Report reported its second annual list of the *Best Diets*, as ranked by a panel of "22 nationally recognized experts in diet, nutrition, obesity, food psychology, diabetes, and heart disease." The expert panel evaluated 28 diets including the well-known Atkins, South Beach Diet, Biggest Loser Diet, and Paleo Diet, and the not so well known Medifast and Cookie diets.

On a sliding scale of 1 to 5, the expert panel rated each diet on ability to "produce short-term and long-term weight loss, its nutritional completeness, its safety, and its potential for preventing and managing diabetes and heart disease." While the Ornish Diet came out on top for best heart-healthy diet and Weight Watchers got the nod for best weight-loss, the DASH diet, which stands for Dietary Approaches to Stop Hypertension, took home the gold. Much to the dismay of its growing legions of supporters, the Paleo Diet was not popular among the panel experts, coming in at the back of the pack (see how it favored in questions 9 and 10 below).

The U.S. News & World Report Best Diets report got a lot of play in the media, and judging by the thousands who commented in a YES or NO to liking a particular diet on the list, the public is paying attention. The overall winner, the DASH diet, is built on the theory that a low-fat, low sodium strategy with a hint towards calorie restriction is the healthiest way to go. But is it?

Given the avalanche of peer-reviewed studies linking the human microbiome (all our microbes and their genes) to everything from obesity, type 2 diabetes, heart disease, some cancers, autoimmune diseases, IBD - and the list goes on - it might be interesting to get the opinion of microbiologist of what might constitute a healthier dietary strategy, but from the view of the microbiome.

What if many of our acute and chronic diseases are an imbalance with the microbial world? While it's a big what if, the 16 papers recently published as part of the Human Microbiome Project - not to mention hundreds of other papers published in the last few years alone - suggest that we need to start rethinking what makes us sick. Given what might be the proverbial writing on the wall, it's probably not much of a stretch to suggest that dietary and lifestyle advice, which currently comes from a physicians, general practitioners and registered dietitians, will likely come from a microbiologist or related specialist working with the microbiome in the very near future. Or at a minimum, we are going to see GPs and RDs with increased training in "medical ecology" and evolutionary principles.

So with this in mind, I created a dietary questionnaire

(below) and sent it to microbiologists who work with diet, disease, metabolism and so on in the context of the microbiome. Some of the researchers I knew, most I did not. And many opted not to participate. In some instances its frowned upon by institutions for their researchers to participate in such surveys. (For those that did, and could, it's much appreciated). It is also acknowledged that some of the questions in the survey minimize the complexity of the interactions that are at play in linking the microbiome to a condition of interest - and that much of our understanding of the role of the microbiome in human disease is preliminary. There was no way around that while trying to keep the questions and answers understandable to a general audience. Its also acknowledged, that while the possibilities associated with changing or altering the microbiome for better health is within reach for some ailments, nobody wants to take the cake out of the oven too soon. So the scientists working in the field are optimistically cautious about their work.

Unlike some of the experts in the U.S. News & World Report survey, I don't think many of the microbiologists have a horse in the race so to speak. They are interested in the microbiome and its modulation and impact on its host (you and me). Not a particular or popular diet or philosophy. This, of course, may be naive and shortcoming of the results presented here. But nevertheless, the microbiologist were all asked to consider the questions and their answers in the context of the microbiome without regard to a "named or labeled" diet plan. For this reason the questions were not about a specific diet plan, as was done in the U.S. News & World Report survey, but more "indirect" questions.

Below are the results from 37 microbiologists who had responded within 24 hours of sending out the survey. It includes researchers from all over the world from major research universities and organizations. Note the respondents were anonymous, as I did not want them to receive a bunch of emails from individuals who may not have agreed with their answers. Again, another shortcoming of the survey, but it is what it is. The survey was limited to 10 questions in all (with several sub questions within questions). Without a doubt, more questions could have been asked and the questions asked could have all been worded differently - so shoot holes in it if you must.

The questions and the average answer on the sliding scale are provided. Brief comments are provided after each question and a take home summary is provided at the end. We would love to get your feedback on this and please share these results with others.

Q1. Does diet play a role in shaping the human gut microbiome?

(1 = strongly disagree and 10 = strongly agree)
Results: 8.9
The question was pretty straightforward and an average answer of 8.9 is consistent with the research that diet modulates gut microbiome composition.

Q2. Do you believe increasing diversity within the gut microbiome is important?

(1 = strongly disagree and 10 = strongly agree)

Results 7.4

The concept of diversity is best understood from an ecological perspective. Since our gut microbiome is an "inner ecosystem," made up of thousands of species, increased species diversity within the microbiome is emerging as an indicator of potentially positive diet and lifestyle choices - and a hallmark of our evolutionary past.

Q3. Do you believe our ancestors had a more diverse inner ecosystem?

(1 = strongly disagree and 10 = strongly agree)

Results 6.4

Given the lifestyle of our ancestors it is hypothesized - though data is lacking - that our ancestral life exposed us to a greater diversity of microorganisms on a daily basis. This, coupled with the lack of antibiotics, which is known to impact diversity in our modern microbiome, suggests that our ancestral microbiome may have been characterized by greater diversity. Again, maybe. Future research is needed.

Q4. Do the following play a role in shaping the human gut microbiome? Sorry for the long list.

(1 = strongly disagree and 10 = strongly agree)

There were several sub questions in this question. Questions were:

Birthing method (c-section vs vaginal): Results 8.3

Length of breast-feeding (months, years): Results 8.0

Early childhood exposure to antibiotics: Results 9.3
Lifetime exposure to antibiotics (all sources): Results 9.2
(Hygiene) Lifetime exposure to animals, soil, etc: Results 9.1
Sodium in diet: Results 3.6
Taking vitamin supplements: Results 3.5
Organic vs conventionally grown vegetables: Results 4.7
Organic vs conventionally raised meat: Results 3.4

Mounting evidence suggests that how you enter this world (c-section *vs* vaginal) and whether or not you are breast-fed, and for how long, may have short and long-term effects on the composition of your microbiome. However, as one of the survey respondents indicated in a comments section, the long-term effects into adult life are "completely unknown." Additional, long-term studies are needed. The idea that early childhood and lifetime exposure to antibiotics from medicine and our food supply is receiving a considerable amount of research attention - given that disruption of the microbiome by antibiotics is well documented. Their long-term roles in things such as obesity are currently being considered. It's clear from the low scores for sodium and vitamin intake, and whether or not you consume organic or conventionally grown foods; the survey respondents do not think that any of these has much of an impact on your gut microbiome.

Q5. Although accessibility by various bacterial groups will vary, do you believe in general that dietary fiber and resistant starch are beneficial for the microbiome?
(1 = strongly disagree and 10 = strongly agree)
Results 8.5

It is widely accepted that dietary fiber and resistant starch serve as substrates for bacteria growth in the large bowel (colon). Increasing the delivery of substrates to the residing bacteria results in greater short chain fatty acid production (SCFA) and reduction in colonic pH - both of which are desirable. And if those substrates include special dietary fiber known as prebiotics, it may also improve gut barrier function.

Q6. Do you believe the current USDA's Dietary Guidelines for Americans were compiled with a clear understanding of the impact of dietary choices on the microbiome?

(1= Probably not, 10= Yes)

Results 1.3

A quick review of the panel of experts assembled to update the 2005 Dietary Guidelines for Americans to the current 2010 guidelines (myPlate), reveals a diverse group of distinguished researchers within their respective fields. But the omission of researchers who work with the gut microbiome is unfortunate. And unless I missed it, neither the 2010 dietary guidelines nor the accompanying 1,375-page report from the Institute of the Office of Medicine, contain the word microbiome anywhere in the text. The respondents to this survey do not think much consideration was given to the microbiome either. Maybe next time.

Q7. Based on current research - and what research might reveal in the future - do you believe the microbiome might play a role in the following

disease/condition?

(1 = strongly disagree and 10 = strongly agree)

There were several sub questions in this question. Questions were:

Colon cancer: Results 9.4

Obesity: Results 8.6

Type 2 diabetes: Results 8.6

Heart Disease: Results 8.3

IBD: Results 9.4

Autoimmune disease in general: Results 8.3

Metabolic diseases in general: Results 9.1

Select other cancers in general: Results 7.8

Autism: Results 5.3

Other cognitive disorders in general: Results 6.2

Gut permeability and systemic inflammation: Results 9.3

The results above were somewhat expected. You can Google the disease + microbiome and access published research associated with each. There is lots of it. For some, like obesity, the role of the gut microbiome is well established, but much work remains to be done. For others, like autism, there are only tantalizing hints that our gut bugs may play a role. With each an underlying genetic susceptibility is required and then an environmental trigger. More often than not, that environmental trigger is diet related. What should be of great interest is the general consensus that is forming around the role of the microbiome and gut permeability - or leaky gut. Once an imbalance (dysbiosis) occurs, be it from diet, antibiotics or so on, a chain reaction occurs and things leak into the bloodstream, which can lead to low-grade inflammation associated with obesity, type 2 diabetes and some other less desirable things. One condition that was inadvertently left off the list was the autoimmune disorder Celiac disease. Mounting research is linking the gut microbiome with the timing and onset of this debilitating disease.

Q8. General diet related questions.

(1= I have no idea, 10= strongly agree)
Would low GI foods be preferable?: Results 5.6
Would a raw food diet be less desirable: Results 4.6
Is a calorie a calorie? Or, is dietary quality more important than qty? Results: 7.5
Does source of protein matter (plant vs animal)? Results: 6.6

As a general rule - again, general - someone who follows a low glycemic diet (low GI) will be consuming more whole foods. Translation: more minimally processed plants. Again, in theory, this would raise the amount of naturally occurring dietary fiber in the diet. This was a round about way of asking "nearly" same question I posed in **Q5** above, which got an 8.5 average response opposed the 5.6 here. Seems the raw food diet is not considered a big deal when it comes to the microbiome – which may have something to do with the idea that cooking increases the energy density of the food item and also cleaves the structure of the plants in such a way that make more of the material available for fermentation (i.e., less may pass out the other end). I threw in the calorie is a calorie question in light of the recent study published in the *Journal of the American Medical Association* that not all calories are created equal. As I was told, the "does the source of the protein matter" question could have probably been worded differently. I can only assume what the respondents thought I was getting at - so the 6.6 is middle of the road to slight agree, but for what I'm not sure. Maybe that plant protein is more interesting if it comes in a package that also delivers some fermentable substrates (fiber) along with it.

Q9. Do you believe a better understanding of the nutritional landscape (and lifestyle) of our ancestors (and remote, traditional communities today) might provide insight into the conditions that selected for our current human-associated microbiome?
(1= strongly disagree, 10= strongly agree)
Results 9.1

A recent study published in the journal *Nature* comparing the gut microbiome of U.S. citizens to individuals living in Malawi and the Amazonas of Venezuela, reveal differences. This study, and others among less westernized populations, suggests that our modern world and its highly processed diet may be changing our microbiome as well. But the jury is still out on whether it's changing for the better or worse. The latter is more likely. Therefore, it may be prudent to better understand the nutritional and ecological landscape that selected for our modern human-associated microbiome.

Q10. Do you believe a high protein-fat diet, so long as it includes a significant amount and diversity of whole plants (fermentation sources) and minimal to no processed carbohydrates, is a strategy for a healthy microbiome?

(1= strongly disagree, 10= strongly agree)
Results 9.1

I threw this question in due to the whippin' that the Paleo Diet got in the U.S. News & World Report survey. The experts ranked it 24th overall. The theory behind the Paleo diet is simple: if our ancestors ate it, you should eat it. If they didn't, you shouldn't either. This means things like grains and dairy are out, and lots of meat and fruits and veggies are in. Even though the data suggest otherwise, some continue to be concerned that the high fat intake may have deleterious effects. In addition, the adherence does not seem to be an issue for the multitudes now following the Paleo lifestyle. While the fat issue may be of concern when it comes to leaky gut and associated inflammation, it's not when that diet includes a significant quantity and diversity of plants, which the diet proponents advocate. At an average score of 9.1, the Paleo Diet is in line with a healthy microbiome.

In summary, I paraphrase Michael Pollan: Eat dirt, not too much, mainly with plants (and meat is ok, even with a little fat on it).

17

IS FOOD TEXTURE MORE IMPORTANT THAN CALORIES IN PREVENTING WEIGHT GAIN?

Is a calorie just a calorie? Whether from a wheat bagel or a Snickers bar, is 300 calories, regardless of the source, just that: 300 calories? The experts say yes. This thought process then leads to the positive-caloric-balance hypothesis as an explanation of weight gain and obesity. In short, eat more calories than your body uses and you will gain weight. Seems logical.

These same researchers will quickly point to the first law of thermodynamics (the law of energy conservation) to bolster a cause and effect that implies that any change in body weight must equal the difference in the amount consumed versus the amount expended (For a brilliant book on the history of this argument see *Good Calories, Bad Calories* by Gary Taubes).

The energy balance equation looks like this:

Change in energy stores = Energy intake − Energy

expenditure

To this day, nearly a century of obesity research has been based on this simple formula. However, most obesity researchers and public health officials rely only on the right side of the equation (Energy intake − Energy expenditure) to explain obesity, conveniently ignoring the left side (Changing in energy stores). These experts correctly assume that a positive caloric balance is associated with weight gain, but they assume without justification that positive caloric balance is the cause of obesity. Any adult female can attest to the role of hormones in weight gain—a gain that is unrelated to caloric balance. This is made clearer during pregnancy; when hormone-driven evolutionary forces promote hunger, weight gain, and lethargy—all to assure that sufficient calories are available for the newborn. This and other misconceptions of weight gain and obesity have lead to over a century of misguided obesity research that continues to this day.

With all due respect to the raw food movement, cooked food just tastes better. And from an evolutionary perspective, the application of heat to our food has played a significant role in the success of our species. But are we cooking our food a little too much?

Cooking makes a food more digestible than the same food without the benefit of cooking. In carbohydrate-rich foods, the application of heat to a moisture-rich food (e.g., a potato) causes hydrogen bonds in the glucose polymers to weaken, causing the tight crystalline structure to loosen and gelatinize. As long as water is present in the food or the cooking environment, the starch will gelatinize. Once consumed, the gelatinized starches are more easily cleaved by our digestive enzymes, thus more digestible. The same process occurs in meats through denaturation of proteins through the application of heat.

From an evolutionary perspective, we may be cooking *some* of our food a tad too much for *cultural* and *culinary* reasons, and in the process affecting some time-honored physiological requirements of the human body—specifically, the role of the stomach in energy balance, satisfaction, and hunger.

It was not that long ago that all of our foods were minimally processed. In short, crunchier, grainier, and definitely less refined. There is no doubt that our ancestors would marvel at the sleek and gelatinized angel hair pasta of today and the pasty softness of a steamed carrot torpedo. While convenient and tasty, our modern processing (in the case of the finely milled flour in the pasta) and cooking techniques ("hyper" steamed veggies) have moved digestion from the stomach to the stovetop. All the extra cooking in our modern lifestyle has slowly eliminated—or at least reduced—the role the human stomach evolved to play in digestion. And herein lies the discordance between our modern lifestyle and its nifty technological tools and cultural preferences, with our evolution-determined physiology and specifically, energy balance.

The carrot-like tuber your ancestors ate either raw or minimally cooked has been replaced by foods with a texture like baby food. This texture comes from weakened glucose polymers caused by the application of super-efficient cooking techniques. By way of example, the modern cooked carrot is easily digested and therefore rapidly moved through the stomach. It's safe to say that modern humans are experiencing some of the fastest rates of gastric emptying in human history. Gone are the days when minimally processed foods stayed in the stomach for two, three, or even four hours. There's no longer a need for food to stay in the stomach; the stovetop started the digestion well ahead of ingestion, greatly speeding the work of gastric enzymes.

This effect is nicely captured in the widely popular Glycemic Index (GI). The GI ranks foods according to their effect on blood glucose levels. High GI foods, like highly processed donuts and sugary soft drinks, cause a rapid rise in blood glucose and subsequent insulin levels. Not good. Foods that are processed less *generally* have a lower GI.

But cooking has a significant and often unappreciated effect on the GI of a food. A raw carrot, which takes some crunching to break down, is transferred to the stomach, where some time-honored digestion takes place in a natural and slow way. Thus, a raw carrot has a low GI (about 16). However, a peeled and boiled carrot is easy to chew and rapidly processed in the stomach, as it has been predigested on the stovetop. This cooked carrot has a higher GI, around 60. This translates to rapid gastric emptying and subsequent rapid absorption—resulting in elevated glucose and insulin levels. Not good.

So what does this have to do with weight gain? Aside from some issues related to elevated levels of insulin in the blood—which has a dramatic impact on fat metabolism — the processed carrot versus the unprocessed carrot is tinkering with some evolutionary processes related to thermogenesis, and may be playing an unrealized role in our national epidemic of obesity. This is nicely demonstrated in an elegant study recently published by Japanese researchers. (Hang in there, almost to the point!)

In this study, a team of Japanese scientists from Kyushu University divided 20 rats into two groups of 10 at four weeks of age. Over the next 22 weeks, both groups ate a nutritionally identical diet of rat chow. However, for one group of rats, the hard-to-chew pellets were injected with a tiny bit of air, making them softer and easier to chew. This is more or less similar to our raw versus steamed carrot discussion above.

The air-injected pellets were more like breakfast cereal and required about half as much force to chew and break down. The hard and the soft pellets were the same in how they were cooked, in their nutrient composition, and in their water content. Based on the "calorie is a calorie" argument and the first law of thermodynamics discussed above, rats reared under identical conditions and consuming the same nutrition should grow at the same rate and size and with the same amount of body fat and overall weight. But they did not.

Even though the rats had identical energy intake throughout the 22-week experiment, the rats, which consumed the soft pellets slowly, become heavier. It was gradual at first, but the rats fed soft pellets weighed about 6% more than the harder pellet eaters and had 30 percent more abdominal fat—enough to be classified as obese. The difference documented was due to the cost of digestion.

Before and after feeding, the researchers measured the

body temperature of each rat. At every meal the rats experienced a rise in body temperature, but the rise was less in the soft pellet group. The difference in temperature was most significant between the groups within an hour of ingesting a meal, when the stomach is churning and secreting. The researchers concluded that the softer diet resulted in obesity simply because it was less costly to digest. Increased heat during digestion burns calories at a faster rate; similar to the weight loss we experience when we're sick with a fever.

We all know that weight gain does not happen over night. It's a slow process that takes place over long periods of time and can fluctuate dramatically. And because this is a slow and gradual process, we also know the body is constantly trying to regulate energy intake to energy expended. The body strives for balance, not an imbalance. This is why you are hungry after vigorous physical exercise; your body wants to replace the calories you just burned. This also explains why a lumberjack needs 5,000 to 8,000 calories a day, but an advertising executive might only need 2,500 or so. If exercise were the answer, then all meter maids would be thin. But they are not.

Weight gain among a given population has more to do with tinkering with evolutionary processes than with sloth or one's willpower. It's uniquely biological. If the experts are correct in that small changes, like 90 minutes of exercise a week or 100 calorie snacks are the answer, then paying attention to the level of processing of our food discussed in this blog should have at least as much merit in fighting the obesity epidemic.

I am not advocating a raw food diet—oh hell no! That's a sure way to guarantee you don't get sufficient nutrients and will surely bore yourself and your loved ones to near death—literally. And raw beef is downright dangerous. I am suggesting that you take a closer look at the amount of processed food you eat. Think, before you steam rice for 15 minutes, that maybe 12 minutes would be enough— making it a little crunchier and therefore a tad harder for your stomach to break down. This will, in turn, elevate your body temperature slightly as your stomach churns and burns calories. You might also consider doing the same with steamed broccoli. In addition, don't cut off and throw away the stalks and eat just the yummy crown. Cut that fiber-rich stalk into thin slices and steam away. By increasing the fiber in your meals, you will also give your stomach a chance to do its job as well.

18

AN EATERS GUIDE TO A HEALTHIER MICROBIOME

"I have 15 cows, how many do you have?" Chief Jambiru asked me.

"How many cows do I have?" I thought. What an odd question. But I shouldn't have thought so, as I had just asked the Chief how many cows he owned.

Turning my bovine query back on me caught me a little off guard and it took me a moment to realize he was not poking fun at me, but seriously wanted know how many cows I owned.

"None at the moment," I said.

So there we sat, in a dry, sandy creek bed high in the rugged mountains of northern Namibia near the Angola border, me cross-legged on one side of the crackling fire and the Chief in a deep squat perched effortlessly on a fist-sized stone on the other side, both thinking to ourselves how curious the other was. *How could I not have any cows!*

I was only the second white man the Chief had ever seen, according to our translator Ziggie. A few years back, the Chief had crossed paths with another white guy hiking in the mountains in search of what I gathered was exotic Aloe Vera plants. Though the translation was a little sketchy. I guess I shouldn't have been surprised when Ziggie verified that a female colleague in our group was the first white woman the Chief had ever laid eyes on.

To be fair, the Chief and his three friends who also squatted effortlessly onto frighteningly small stones in the sand around the fire, along with the twenty or so other men, women and children in his dry-season camp located only a stones throw from our camp fire, were the first mountain Otjhimba I had ever met. It was a number of firsts all around.

As the evening went on and the Southern Cross appeared in the night sky, the smell and sound of fresh meat – a gift from the Chief – sizzled atop hot rocks on the edge of the fire filling the cool night air. I began to wonder if we had found the people I had traveled 8,000 miles to the bottom of the world to locate. Were these the Honey People of the mountains of northern Namibia – one of the last true remaining hunter-gatherer groups in all of southern Africa? The presence of cows, no matter how scrawny – and the distinctive "maaa" of goats in the distance – suggested no. *True* hunter-gatherers do not keep livestock.

Had globalization finally caught up with the Honey People, was I a few years too late, or were we in the wrong dry creek bed, on the wrong mountain, sharing meat with the wrong, though stunningly gracious, people?

I started to do the math. If I was only the second white man and the first was the Aloe Vera hunter, then these could not be the Honey People as I had learned of their whereabouts from a white South African who had spent several days with them back in 2006. That meant I should have been the third white man. Surely the Chief would have remembered *white man number one*.

My trek to the hills of northern Namibia and the meeting with the Chief took place this past summer. I was there because despite piles of peer-reviewed research and major research efforts such as the NIH's massive Human Microbiome Project and similarly large efforts in Europe, we still do not have a good handle on what a 'normal' or 'healthy' gut microbiome looks like. And we may never know. It may be that our modern world of processed foods, antibiotics, fancy indoor plumbing and a wet wipe at every turn, may have forever altered our ancient gut inhabitants. (Remember your gut microbiome is all the microbes in your gut and their genes).

I thought about the Chief and why I had gone to Africa the other day while leaning against my shopping cart at our local grocery store – trying to decide what I should eat that night. More specifically, what should I feed my gut bugs. I spent a lot of time over the last few years pouring over every microbiome-related study showing how diet (and lifestyle) shift the composition of our gut microbiome. We know that most of us have more or less hundreds (if not a lot more) species of bacteria in our gut – some of whom are permanent members who numbers go up and down and others are more transient (just passing through as they say).

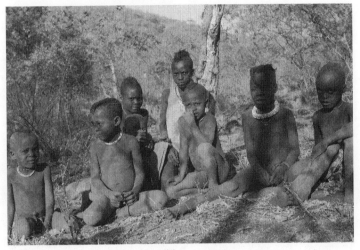

Otjhimba kids in northern Namibia.

There are countless studies showing that if you feed humans or mice either a low fat, high fiber, or All-American westernized diet, the composition of the bacteria shifts (some species/genus/phyla go up in number, some go down). These experiments reveal that you can start with one diet, check the composition of the bacteria using DNA techniques, then change the diet for a period of time, measure again, and then shift the diet back to the original (baseline), then analyze the bacteria at the end. Throughout this roller coaster of diet shifts (sound familiar?), the bacterial communities shift as well. Depending on the study, the shifts occur at higher phylogenic levels (like shifts in the phyla Firmicutes and Bacteroidetes), but in some studies shifts at lower genus and species levels are apparent.

In either case, we can say with some level of certainty that dietary input shapes the composition of our gut microbial community. But should we be worried that our gut microbial communities shift around as a function of what we eat and if so, which composition (or 'state' as the ecologists like to say), should we be aiming for? That is the million-dollar question.

We know that someone who takes antibiotics can dramatically shift their gut microbes. When this happens, the diversity of the gut microbial 'ecosystem' also declines. When diversity declines – among other things – the individual is susceptible to secondary infection. The most talked about secondary infection is by *Clostridium difficile*, or C. Diff for short. The scorched earth outcome of many broad-spectrum antibiotics is analogous to spraying poison all over your backyard plants and grass and waiting to see what grows back. In the case of your gut ecosystem – just like in your yard – invasive and maybe some not-so-good species (microbes in the case of your gut and some funky weeds in your yard) carve out a niche in the available gut/yard landscape.

From this perspective – gut microbial communities as ecosystems – the ecological principles of diversity and resilience start to help you think about how to fortify your gut against not only invaders that seek to do you harm (also think about E. Coli and others), but also about nurturing a diverse community within your gut that provides what ecologists call 'ecosystem services.' In the case of your gut bugs, the services they provide include harvesting energy from otherwise useless nutrients like dietary fiber, pathogen resistance through a number of mechanisms, synthesizing vitamins, assisting in the maintenance of the mucosal barrier that lines in the inside of your intestinal tract – which helps regulate immune response and reduce leaky gut – and the list goes on. In short, when your gut ecosystem shifts as a result of a perturbation – like an insult from an antibiotic, drug, or a shift in your diet maybe – then your equilibrium is out of balance and you tip towards an unstable state which may open you up to disease.

Some interesting studies in mice and humans have shown that a high fat diet can shift your gut microbes which in turn has the knock on effect of low-grade inflammation as measured by circulating levels (in your blood) of a plasma endotoxin known as lipopolysaccharide (LPS). LPS is the primary structural component of the outer membrane of Gram-negative bacteria found in the gut. So how can shifting your gut microbes cause an increase of LPS in your blood? Turns out, the high fat diet reduces (shifts) the levels of Bifidobacterium. These particular bacteria are known to produce short-chain fatty acids (butyrate, propionate and lactate) as a byproduct of fermenting things like dietary fiber. When their numbers go down – as with a high fat diet – the amount of short-chain fatty acids (SCFA) go down as well. These SCFAs are known to improve gut barrier function (think leaky gut) through a number of mechanisms.

So, in this 'one example,' if you change your diet (higher fat in this case) you reduce your SCFA production – which is an ecosystem service provided by your microbes – then your gut starts to leak and things that do not belong in your blood start showing up (LPS) causing low-grade inflammation (the lab coats call it endotoxemia) which has been linked to insulin resistance, type 2 diabetes and obesity (see *Can a high-fat Paleo Diet cause obesity and diabetes article*). It's interesting to note, that its not the fat *per se* that causes the Bifidobacterium to shift downward in abundance and thus cause a leaky gut, but the reduction of fermentable substrates. That's is, you cut off the Bifido's food supply and thus they slow down the SCFA production - which is protective. As the famous Rajin Cajun James Carville might say, "It's the Fiber stupid."

So what should you eat to improve the diversity and possible resilience of your gut microbiome to reduce the risk of invading pathogens, unnecessary inflammation, leaky gut and so forth? Nobody really knows for sure and the answer is likely different for different age groups and populations. But at a minimum, you want that ecosystem service of SCFAs to keep churning along at high levels - so eat as many plants a week as you can (30-50 is a good number to shoot for - keep track and see how you do) - that is, keep the fiber (non-starch polysaccharides, resistant starch etc) flowing to your colon. And maybe cut back a bit on the easy to digest and hyper-cooked and processed foods - letting your stomach do a little extra-somatic work every now and then. Maybe even open a window every now and then, and for god's sake, get your hands and food a little dirty. But if we ever hope to get a better handle on what a 'normal' or 'healthy' gut (or skin, oral etc for that matter) microbiome looks like, we will need to look at less westernized populations who are still undergoing the epidemiological transitions most of us have already undergone.

Getting a larger sample of westernized gut microbiomes is necessary as well and the reason we launched the

American Gut project – to crowd source 10,000 gut microbiomes across the diversity that is the American Gut. It is also the reason I was trekking in the mountains of northern Namibia. With detailed dietary and lifestyle data and the resulting microbiomes from the American Gut project, we will be able to see patterns not otherwise possible in smaller groups of people. By comparing this data set to more traditional societies – the microbial Noah's Arks I like to think of them as – we might get a glimpse of how the process of village to urban life shifted and altered our ancient gut microbiome to its current – and very possibly – persistently perturbed state.

I will be headed back to that mountaintop in the next few months to see the Chief again, and explore a few new valleys and ridge tops in the hopes of locating these ghosts of our ancestral past. And hopefully they will agree to help.

19

BIO SIZE ME, PLEASE

Fresh off her much-applauded announcement of important changes to the government-subsidized school lunch program, Michelle Obama has been sweeping the nation promoting the second anniversary of "Let's Move" by judging an elementary school cooking challenge with Top Chefs, dancing the Platypus Walk at Disney Orlando, and doing push ups with Ellen DeGeneres. It's uplifting to see so much attention finally being showered upon getting healthy. Now all she needs to do is take her vegetable cart over to the USDA and run it over the newly introduced *MyPlate* a few times. If we ever want to stem the tide of obesity and chronic disease in this country, and we cannot exercise our way out of this problem, we are going to need to break a few plates.

In summer of 2011 Michelle Obama, book-ended by Agriculture Secretary Tom Vilsack and surgeon general Dr. Regina Benjamin, unveiled the government's latest effort to get Americans to make healthier choices. Out was the much-loathed Food Pyramid and in was the snazzy *MyPlate* with its visual portioning. Fruits and veggies got half the plate.

Though much of the media yawned, health professionals in general agreed the new visual direction of a plate was an improvement and acknowledged that the accompanying *Dietary Guidelines for Americans*, which are mandated by Congress to be updated every five years, were also an improvement.

At the unveiling of the new *MyPlate*, the First Lady proclaimed if the filled plate looks like the symbol, with lots of fruits and vegetables, "then we're good, it's as simple as that." But we are not good. And for the three decades the government has been handing down dietary recommendations, we have been getting sicker, wider, and more medicated. And even though the *5-A-Day* message has been promoted endlessly, our national consumption of fruits and veggies has been flat to almost non-existent for nearly four decades (see chapter *If only vegetables smelled as good as bacon*)

By any measure, dietary advice handed down by the USDA (and Department of Health and Human Services) has not been as effective as hoped, and by some measures, actually harmful. The decade's long push to lower fat consumption, a recommendation that was *never* based on sound evidence, resulted in a devastating increase in processed carbohydrates and likely played a causal role in the increase of metabolic disease and its handmaiden, obesity.

Government-sponsored dietary advice matters as 32 million school lunches are formulated on these recommendations, not to mention a dizzying number of federal food programs ranging from the military to prisons.

So what are we to do? History tells us the strategy isn't working no matter how big of a piece we carve out for fruits and veggies on *MyPlate*, and continuing to think we will get a different outcome is, well, by Albert Einstein's definition, insanity. A good place to (re)start, aside from moving the responsibility of developing these guidelines out from under the USDA, whose mission is to promote agriculture by the way, would be to bring the guidelines in line with extraordinary advances in genomics, microbiology and medicine that are unwinding in front of our eyes.

The current dietary advice ignores the biological fact that 90% of the cells in the human body are not even human; they are microbial. Yet, we design dietary advice that completely ignores the symbiotic and sometimes pathogenic relationship we evolved with these evolutionary hitchhikers. Though our bodies are covered in microbial life, the far reaches of our gut harbors trillions of members who have become so important to our health and well-being they are collectively referred to as the "forgotten organ."

The diversity of this forgotten organ, known as the microbiome, rivals the most diverse ecosystems on earth, our inner ecosystem. Advances in genomic research in the last decade have made it possible to unravel just how important maintaining balance, or symbiosis, with our microbiome is. Changes in the composition of the microbiome, or even single members, are now known to play a role in ailments as diverse as obesity, diabetes, cancer,

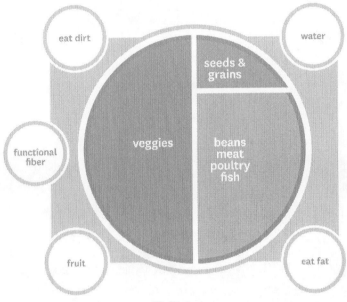

BioPlate.

atherosclerosis, inflammatory bowel disease, and a great many neurological disorders. Further, tiny viruses that embed themselves inside members of our microbiome may play a part in a great many more diseases of humanity.

A great many factors including genetics, age, sex, and diet influence the microbiome. However, of these, diet is the easiest to influence. Astonishingly, researchers have determined that the entire human population can be grouped into roughly three groups based on the composition of the microbiome – this, in spite of age, weight, sex or nationality.

What we need is a *BioPlate*, not *MyPlate*. We need dietary recommendations that recognize humans are amalgam of human and microbial cells – a super organism. This *BioPlate* would down play fructose-bearing fruits, moving them off the plate to the treat or dessert section, where they belong, resulting in half the plate (or more) being vegetables. And when we add in a healthy dose of beans and legumes (sorry my Paleo Diet friends), and dial up the fat via nuts and the like, we have a plate dominated by plants. These same plants will provide a diverse and rich nutrient base that our microbiome evolved on and our modern lifestyle has all but removed, resulting in imbalance (dysbiosis). The *Bioplate* would also shrink the grains section (a lot), highlight whole grains, and promote more diversity. Meat is not out, far from it. Just consume it smarter. The *BioPlate* would also suggest we spend a little more time at the Farmers Market, buying and consuming a few more plants covered in microbial-laden soil (see chapter *Farmer's Market Rx*). Our squeaky clean food supply of triple-washed leafy greens and carrots shaped like bullets, has removed health giving microorganisms and left our immune system unchallenged and thus over reactive.

The science to better health is staring us in the face; we just need to pay attention. The prestigious journal *Science* picked the microbiome as one of the breakthrough's of 2011, acknowledging the literally hundreds of scientific articles published on the subject in the last year alone. This is disheartening when you consider that the USDA's 95 page 2010 *Dietary Guidelines for Americans* and the Institute of Medicine's accompanying 1,375 page report on dietary reference intakes did not mention the word microbiome. Not once.

The time is now. We need the First Lady to drag her

vegetable cart over to the NIH-funded Human Microbiome Project, a $160M undertaking that is unraveling the correlation between changes in the human microbiome and human health, and ask for a briefing. We can no longer allow industry, single ingredients, or special interests dictate the future health of America. Not to sound cavalier, but nutrition and disease is this generation's civil rights movement; let's start treating it accordingly.

20

A WINDOW INTO YOUR HEALTH

Sitting on the floor of a traditional Himba hut in northern Namibia this past summer, I found myself staring at a peculiar hand-sized hole located about halfway up the curved wall thinking to myself, "what could be the purpose of such a small opening?" Turns out, it was the sole portal to the outside world – at least when the tiny three foot door was closed. It was a window – but why so small?

In the absence of available panes of glass to the Himba in this arid region, I reasoned that if they had made it bigger, say two feet by two feet, the rain would trickle in. It would, not to mention, serve as an invite for an enumerable number of crawling and flying pests. The keep-the-rain-out logic started to make the most sense when I realized the gaps and openings surrounding the closed door hardly kept even the largest of nature's pests – save a goat – from entering the home.

After spending a few hours in this village near the Angola border – we had come to ask permission to take

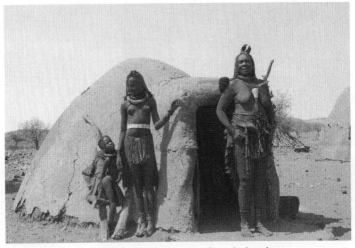

Himba family in northern Namibia near Angola border.

swabs of their homes to characterize the microbes they
shared their living quarters with – I started to appreciate
why a single, tiny window was all that was needed in any
Himba hut. As with most traditional societies and
throughout human evolution, people lived outside. Cooking,
socializing and a big chunk of sleeping during the warmer
and less rainy part of the year, was done outside. Adding
more or larger windows to a space that was only used
sparingly – and even then mainly at night – and the need to
look outside and gain some knowledge of what was going
on or to appreciate the "outdoors" was less important. It
was likely dark and you got your full of "outside" having
spent the majority of your day in it.

Add to this those gaping holes around a door that was
more of a suggestion than an obstacle to entry, and the floor
and wall plaster made of cow dung, you quickly become
conscious of the fact that for 99.99% of human history the

outside was always part of the inside, and at no moment during our day were we ever really separated from nature. This ecological reality makes our modern built environment of hermitically sealed lives of ventilated and filtered air and large pane glass windows seem at odds with the natural order of things. Keeping the outside out does have its advantages – protection from the elements and decreasing your chances of being eaten by a predator in some areas among them. But biologists who study the diversity and composition of the built environment microbiome are starting to think maybe we have walled off and filtered out a little too much of the outside – at least from a microbial perspective.

In urban settings, A National Activity Survey found that between enclosed buildings and vehicles, humans spend a whopping 90% of their lives indoors. Researchers who study the ecology of built spaces from the University of Oregon wanted to know how the airborne microbial life differed in spaces that were either naturally vented through open windows or mechanically ventilated (i.e., central heating and air) and how the microbial environment might impact human health. Since hospitals are both a place of healing and where one might acquire a secondary infection as well, they set up special BioSamplers in various patient rooms at the Providence Milwaukie Hospital in Milwaukie, Oregon.

Using the BioSampler, which draws air through two liquid impingers filled with sterile water and thus traps the dust, pollen and attached microbes, they set up measuring stations in rooms 1) vented 'naturally' through open windows; 2) mechanically vented rooms and; 3) on the roof of the hospital near the air intake for the ventilating system. They also measured things like air temperature, humidity and amount of airflow through the various rooms.

Using high-throughput sequencing of the bacterial 16S rRNA genes of the bacteria captured in the water, they were able to measure the abundance of bacteria as well as species diversity. Between the three environments (mechanically ventilated, window ventilated, and rooftop outside) the airborne bacterial cell density was roughly between 500,000 and 2.5M cells per cubic meter of air sucked through the BioSamplers. Interestingly, the density of cells between these three different environments did not vary significantly. That is, the abundance. However, the highest *diversity* of bacteria was recorded outside, on the rooftop, with the lowest diversity recorded indoors in the mechanically ventilated rooms.

Interestingly, the mechanically ventilated rooms had the greatest *relative abundance* of potential pathogenic bacteria, when compared to either window ventilated rooms or the rooftop outside. In addition, both indoor settings (mechanical and window) also contained bacteria floating in the air that are known to be associated with humans (our regular bugs). Neither the potential pathogenic or human-associated bacteria recorded in both indoor settings were observed in any great abundance from the outdoor samples. The outdoor samples were dominated by bacteria known to occur in soil and water. These soil and water bacteria were "relatively rare or absent indoors" according to the researchers.

The study is fascinating in that it demonstrates how much architectural design and our modern lifestyle changes the microbial ecology of our surroundings. In the case of the Himba, inside is just like the outside – and so it has been for nearly all of human existence. Mechanically ventilated rooms, with filters and return air registers, have an ecologically distinct set of microbes than that found outside on the rooftop. Turns out, the window ventilated rooms have microbial communities somewhere in the middle between outside and those mechanically vented rooms. Also, the outdoor air – though dominated by bacteria found in soil and water – demonstrated a greater diversity of overall bacteria than either indoor setting.

The most important finding of this study is that both indoor environments were dominated by human commensals (known to occur on humans) and known pathogens. The researchers also found that airflow rates through the room had a significant impact on the "pathogen load" of the room. That is, as the air moved in and out of the room via the mechanical ventilation or the natural airflow, the pathogen load was diluted down. It also appeared that temperature and humidity impacted bacterial community composition of the indoor settings as well.

At the moment, while the researchers can rule out the outdoor air as a significant source for the pathogenic and human-associated commensals measured in the rooms, the actual source of these microbial species is not certain, but likely comes from patients and others in the hospital as well as various surfaces – all pushed along with rising and falling temperature and humidity.

Though the researchers did not find any appreciable differences in the pathogen load between mechanical and naturally ventilated rooms, they did note that airflow reduces that load. They also suggest, "that reducing direct contact with the outdoor environment may not always be an optimal design strategy for bacterial pathogen management." In other words, current architects and engineers design buildings for comfort by controlling light, temperature, humidity and airflow – but in the future should consider the management of microbial community as well

Though the researchers do not elaborate on why we should *not* reduce our exposure to the outside, they are implying that "increasing" exchange and airflow with the outside and its soil and water dominated microbial communities may not only reduce the pathogen load even further – and serve as a more economic and ecological friendly way to think about built environments – but reintroduce us to some Old Friends that our transition from village to urban life have scrubbed away.

Seems Florence Nightingale may be more correct than knowable at the time when she said over 150 years ago that open windows were the hallmark of a healthy hospital ward.

Think I will open that window now.

21

DESERT DRIFTING WITH CODY "BAREFOOT" LUNDIN

According to the World Health Organization, key causes of hunger are natural disasters, conflict, poverty, poor agricultural infrastructure and over-exploitation of the environment. I would add to that list spending a week in the high desert of Arizona with Discovery Channel's *Dual Survivor* star Cody "Barefoot" Lundin.

Billed as no ordinary weeklong survival course, Cody's Desert Drifter is designed to "strip you of everything you thought you needed in the wilderness." And in my case, that also meant missing the fine print on the course paperwork I filled out to join this wandering band that would have allowed me a small bag of GORP (granola, oats, raisins, and peanuts) to tide me over as we chased crickets and rabbits for food in northern Arizona. Hunger set in early for me.

As hungry as I was in those first days of calorie burning hikes in extreme temperatures and rough terrain, and an all night march in near freezing temps (shivering burns a large amount of calories), I was faintly comforted by the knowledge that the progressive effects of heat and hypothermia were more likely to kill me than my hunger pangs. With no blankets and a strict "no fire" rule in those first few days, I was left to snippets of communal body heat when we kind of slept and what nourishment I could forage from a landscape that moved quickly under our feet. We were a tribe of nine, drifting now, and the do more with less mantra of the *Aboriginal Living Skills School*, founded by our barefoot leader, began to sink in.

After 48 hours of one extreme survival scenario after another and no sleep, I really began appreciating fine print as my body sucked energy stored from my adipose tissue (aka body fat) and began sipping my strategic energy reserves of glycogen from my liver. My system was struggling to feed my brain and its ability to execute the simplest of cognitive tasks – like putting one foot in front of the other, and completing Cody's primitive skills modules, which also required the dual survival skill of channeling my ancestors with one side of my starved brain and calling up my genetically coded ability to complete fine motor skills with the other. Just another day in the life of our ancient genome, but a rude awakening to a system accustomed to quick energy inputs from a modern nutritional landscape dotted with Chipotle's and 24-hour Circle K's.

The course was designed to beat you down, and beat you down it did. But the one thing that helped me through those first few days – and the remainder of the weeklong survival course for that matter – was my understanding of the

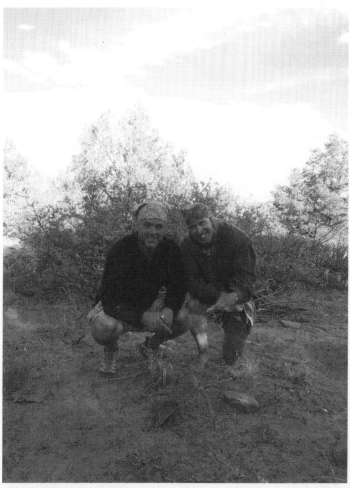

The author and Cody Lundin with a newly constructed Paiute Deadfall (vertical stone).

ancient bioreactor deep in my gut. Nearly five feet in length, the human colon and its trillions of resident bacteria have the ability to generate calories from almost any plant matter, no matter how nutrient-poor that matter may be.

Like the fermentation that takes place in the various stomach chambers of cows, goats etc., the gut bacteria breaks down undigested plant material through various processes and produces byproducts such as short chain fatty acids, which are then absorbed into the body and utilized by the muscles and organs as energy. Depending on the type of undigested plant material (e.g., resistant starch, cellulose, hemicelluloses, inulin, pectins [aka dietary fiber]), the gut bacteria can convert 1 gram of plant matter into as much as 1 to 1.5 calories. Not bad when you consider that the straight-up digestible carbohydrates available, say, in a slice of bread, convert as 1 gram ingested to 4 calories. In other words, bacteria are the reason horses, cows, deer and similar critters can extract enough calories from blades of grass.

So throughout those first few days I literally grazed as we whisked along, grabbing handfuls of green grass, wild flowers, not so tasty berries, and anything that I could choke down. These handfuls of green matter were broken down by my commensal bacteria and turned into calories. Though it was difficult to calculate, I probably generated 300-400 much-needed calories a day from my new trail diet (but likely burned 6-10,000 calories a day). In order to generate even a modest 1,500 to 2,000 calories from the trail diet, I would have had to literally chew all day, and probably locate more energy dense plants (e.g., root foods) that also contained some straight up carbohydrates and starches. We did eventually eat our way into some nutritious stands of cattails – once Cody allowed us the comfort of fire days into the Desert Drifting to cook them.

As with other plant eaters, our earliest of ancestors relied on gut bioreactors to extract calories from otherwise undigested foods. While our colons make up a smaller percentage of our overall gut system today, our ancestors relied on the colonic bioreactor to generate calories from twigs, leaves, flowering plant parts and so on – similar to our tree swinging cousins. But as the quality of our diet improved – through technology and ultimately the advent of fire – the requirement of our bioreactor decreased and therefore its overall size. Even though our colons and their bioreactor function remain a significant part of our gut systems, our modern diet hardly delivers the fermentation products down the pipe as it once did – as I experienced during my week of foraging across the landscape. And there in lays possibly the biggest unappreciated health crisis facing our modern society today.

With a reduction in the consumption of undigested plant parts – to say nothing of the reduction in diversity of plants – we have literally stopped using the calorie-generating bioreactors handed down to us by our ancestors, and in the process created an imbalance in our microbiota that evolved within our gut ecosystem. By not receiving a steady supply and diversity of plant parts (again, fiber), the bacteria living in our guts cannot do their evolutionary job and fight off invading pathogens by increasing acidity, and therefore compete for nutrients and niches in order to flourish along the colonic wall.

The existence of residential microbiota is ancient, providing evidence of the co-evolution of bacteria and animals. In the case of humans, we are endowed with a *specific* set of bacteria at birth and our life history pushes and pulls that balance on a daily basis. Though there is poorly defined variation among human populations, there exists a genome-specific set of players that are significantly influenced by diet.

Rapid changes in diet in our post-modern era are predictably producing different diseases. In short, changes in human ecology equals changes in our microbiota. Add to this the astonishing increases in Caesarean sections that limit perinatal transfer of maternal microflora, which is further confounded by the replacement of mothers milk with formula – which creates an imbalance in natural, indigenous flora.

Advances in molecular and genomic techniques confirm the role of infection in an increasing number of acute and chronic diseases, made more likely by diet and lifestyle-induced imbalance. Disease was heavy on my mind as I drug my weakened body from one cattle tank to another to scoop stagnant, muddied and often dead animal-laden water. But unlike my GORP-eating fine-print-reading colleagues, my steady but limited diet of grass blades and flowers meant my microbiota was bolstered for anything that may have slipped past the iodine drops.

While the biggest threat I faced was diarrhea from bad water, I wouldn't have experienced the impact for a day – or even longer. In fact, the connection between "dirty" water and diarrhea was not made until the 1800s. This same delay from infection to symptom is what delayed acceptance of infectious causation of other vector-borne diseases such as malaria – transmitted by mosquitoes.

But what if many of the chronic diseases plaguing us

today, like heart disease, breast cancer, colon cancer, diabetes and Alzheimer's, all in fact could be ascribed to infectious causation? What if these terrible diseases had a more acute phase, would we then recognize them as the result of infection? Is the lag time between infection and manifestation that characterizes a particular chronic disease shifting our medical attention away from the obvious? I think medical professionals who ignore infectious causation of many of the big chronic killers today will look as myopic to medical historians in 20-30 years from now as the researchers who dismissed infectious causation for pneumonia, chicken pox, and diarrhea did not that long ago.

As we rounded out our desert drifter week we did finally get to enjoy some freshly gathered crawfish from the Verde River along with some crispy grasshoppers roasted on a stick. This was made all the more enjoyable by the fact that I, and everything I ate, was covered in dirt teaming with natural microorganisms with whuch my ancestors had long ago forged a symbiotic relationship. Dirt is good. I never felt so alive.

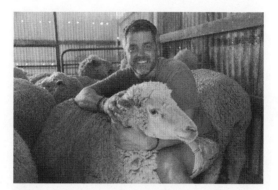

ABOUT THE AUTHOR

Jeff Leach is the Founder of the Human Food Project. His opinions on health and nutrition have appeared as Op-ed articles in the *New York Times, San Francisco Chronicle, Sydney Morning Herald* and his peer-reviewed research has been published in the *British Journal of Nutrition, European Journal of Clinical Nutrition, BioScience and Microflora, Journal of Archaeological Science, Public Health Nutrition* and many others. He lives in New Orleans – but hopes to spend more time in Africa.

NOTES

1   *Americans   report   being:*   Gallup   poll
    http://www.gallup.com/poll/127487/environmental-
    movement-endures-less-consensus.aspx

1   *Human Microbiome Project:* http://www.hmpdacc.org/

2   *predict with 90% accuracy:* Knights, D., Parfrey, L. W.,
    Zaneveld, J., Lozupone, C. & Knight, R. Human-
    Associated Microbial Signatures: Examining Their
    Predictive Value. *Cell host & microbe* **10**, 292-296 (2011).

2   *Staggering number of ailments:* Cho, I. & Blaser, M. J. The
    human microbiome: at the interface of health and
    disease. *Nat Rev Genet* **13**, 260-270 (2012).

2   *Tangled history:* Willett, W. C. & Ludwig, D. S. The 2010
    Dietary Guidelines — The Best Recipe for Health?
    New England Journal of Medicine **365**, 1563-1565,
    doi:doi:10.1056/NEJMp1107075 (2011).

3   *global sustainability agenda:* Reconnecting to the Biosphere
    http://www.earthsystemgovernance.org/publication/f
    olke-carl-reconnecting-biosphere

3   *Researchers   recently   discovered:*   Hanski,   I.   *et   al.*
    Environmental biodiversity, human microbiota, and
    allergy are interrelated. *Proceedings of the National Academy
    of Sciences* **109**, 8334-8339, doi:10.1073/
    pnas.1205624109 (2012).

4   *rewilding our surroundings:* See the excellent book *The
    Wildlife of our Bodies* by Rob Dunn.

4   *the sea-going microbes:* Valentine, D. L. *et al.* Dynamic
    autoinoculation and the microbial ecology of a deep

water hydrocarbon irruption. *Proceedings of the National Academy of Sciences*, doi:10.1073/pnas.1108820109 (2012).

5   *studies in animals*: Turnbaugh, P. J., Backhed, F., Fulton, L. & Gordon, J. I. Diet-induced obesity is linked to marked but reversible alterations in the mouse distal gut microbiome. *Cell Host Microbe* **3**, 213-223 (2008).

5   *climate scientists have:* Anderson, K. & Bows, A. A new paradigm for climate change. *Nature Clim. Change* **2**, 639-640 (2012).

5   *does not register*: Markowitz, E. M. & Shariff, A. F. Climate change and moral judgement. *Nature Clim. Change* **2**, 243-247 (2012).

6   *been recently found*: Smillie, C. S. *et al.* Ecology drives a global network of gene exchange connecting the human microbiome. *Nature* **480**, 241-244 (2011).

7   *team of researchers*: Felton, A. M. *et al.* Protein content of diets dictates the daily energy intake of a free-ranging primate. *Behavioral Ecology* **20**, 685-690, doi:10.1093/beheco/arp021 (2009)

8   *protein leverage hypothesis*: Simpson, S. J. & Raubenheimer, D. Obesity: the protein leverage hypothesis. *Obes Rev* **6**, 133-142 (2005).

17   *Research comparing the*: Ley, R. E. *et al.* Evolution of Mammals and Their Gut Microbes. *Science* **320**, 1647-1651, doi:10.1126/science.1155725 (2008).

17   *Deeper shotgun sequencing*: Muegge, B. D. *et al.* Diet Drives Convergence in Gut Microbiome Functions Across Mammalian Phylogeny and Within Humans. *Science* **332**,

970-974, doi:10.1126/science.1198719 (2011).

21 *the journal Nature*: Hehemann, J.-H. *et al.* Transfer of carbohydrate-active enzymes from marine bacteria to Japanese gut microbiota. *Nature* **464**, 908-912, (2010).

27 *site of Ohalo II*: Weiss, E., Wetterstrom, W., Nadel, D. & Bar-Yosef, O. The broad spectrum revisited: Evidence from plant remains. *Proceedings of the National Academy of Sciences of the United States of America* **101**, 9551-9555, doi:10.1073/pnas.0402362101 (2004).

27 *aborigines are known*: Brand-Miller, J. C. & Holt, S. H. Australian aboriginal plant foods: a consideration of their nutritional composition and health implications. *Nutr Res Rev* **11**, 5-23 (1998).

28 *ancient foraging reveals*: Jeff D. Leach and Kristin D. Sobolik (2010). High dietary intake of prebiotic inulin-type fructans in the prehistoric Chihuahuan Desert. British Journal of Nutrition, 103, pp 1558-1561.

30 *Dozens of peer-reviewed studies*: Roberfroid, M. *et al.* Prebiotic effects: metabolic and health benefits. *Br J Nutr* **104** (2010)

33 *recent WHO report*: Lumbiganon, P. *et al.* Method of delivery and pregnancy outcomes in Asia: the WHO global survey on maternal and perinatal health 2007?08. *The Lancet* **375**, 490-499 (2010)

33 *With rates rising*: http://www.cdc.gov/nchs/data/databriefs/db35.htm

34 *studies of birthing*: Dominguez-Bello, M. G. *et al.* Delivery mode shapes the acquisition and structure of the initial microbiota across multiple body habitats in newborns.

Proceedings of the National Academy of Sciences, doi:10.1073/pnas.1002601107 (2010).

34 *According to Finnish researchers*: http://www.smh.com.au/national/health/csection-babies-at-higher-risk-of-obesity-20120317-1vc22.html

34 *study of 284 infants:* Huh, S. Y. *et al.* Delivery by caesarean section and risk of obesity in preschool age children: a prospective cohort study. *Archives of Disease in Childhood*, doi:10.1136/archdischild-2011-301141 (2012).

34 *rates of asthma*: Bager, P., Wohlfahrt, J. and Westergaard, T. (2008), Caesarean delivery and risk of atopy and allergic disesase: meta-analyses. Clinical & Experimental Allergy, 38: 634–642.

34 *the CDC reports*: http://www.cdc.gov/breastfeeding/data/reportcard.htm

35 *but indigestible oligosaccharides*: Boehm, G. & Stahl, B. Oligosaccharides from Milk. *The Journal of nutrition* **137**, 847S-849S (2007).

35 *their 18ʰ birthday*: Blaser, M. Antibiotic overuse: Stop the killing of beneficial bacteria. *Nature* **476**, 393-394 (2011).

36 *the microbial garden*: http://www.nytimes.com/2012/06/19/science/studies-of-human-microbiome-yield-new-insights.html?_r=1

37 *journal Public Health Nutrition*: Geoffrey Cannon (2007). Out of the Box. Public Health Nutrition, 10, pp 111-114.

40 *the modern Hunza*: Vlahchev, T. & Zhivkov, Z. [Hunza -

138

a healthy and a long living people]. *Asklepii* **15**, 96-97 (2002).

46 *and Lactobacillus, specifically*: Cashman, K. Prebiotics and calcium bioavailability. *Curr Issues Intest Microbiol* **4**, 21-32 (2003)

48 *World Health Organization:* http://www.who.int/foodsafety/publications/fs_management/en/probiotics.pdf

49 *As for prebiotics*: Marcel Roberfroid et al. (2010). Prebiotic effects: metabolic and health benefits. British Journal of Nutrition, 104, pp S1-S63.

50 *$21M fine leeved*: http://www.usatoday.com/money/industries/food/2010-12-15-dannon-misleading-claims-activa-danactive_N.htm

52 *the Hygiene Hypothesis*: Rook, G. A. Hygiene hypothesis and autoimmune diseases. *Clin Rev Allergy Immunol* **42**, 5-15 (2012).

70 *researchers discovered that*: Redman, R. S., Sheehan, K. B., Stout, R. G., Rodriguez, R. J. & Henson, J. M. Thermotolerance Generated by Plant/Fungal Symbiosis. *Science* **298**, 1581, (2002).

70 *those same researchers*: Rodriguez, R. J. *et al.* Stress tolerance in plants via habitat-adapted symbiosis. *Isme J* **2**, 404-416 (2008).

70 *other plants as well*: Redman, R. S. *et al.* Increased Fitness of Rice Plants to Abiotic Stress Via Habitat Adapted Symbiosis: A Strategy for Mitigating Impacts of Climate Change. *PloS one* **6**, (2011).

75 *study by researchers*: Ravussin, E., Valencia, M. E.,

Esparza, J., Bennett, P. H. & Schulz, L. O. Effects of a Traditional Lifestyle on Obesity in Pima Indians. *Diabetes Care* **17**, 1067-1074, (1994).

85 *News & World Report:* http://health.usnews.com/best-diet

107 *large efforts in Europe:* http://www.metahit.eu/

110 *the levels of Bifidobacterium:* Cani, P. D. *et al.* Metabolic Endotoxemia Initiates Obesity and Insulin Resistance. *Diabetes* **56**, 1761-1772, doi:10.2337/db06-1491 (2007).

121 *National Activity Survey:* Klepeis, N. E. *et al.* The National Human Activity Pattern Survey (NHAPS): a resource for assessing exposure to environmental pollutants. *J Expo Anal Environ Epidemiol* **11**, 231-252 (2001).

121 *ecology of built spaces:* Kembel, S. W. *et al.* Architectural design influences the diversity and structure of the built environment microbiome. *Isme J* **6**, 1469-1479 (2012)

126 *Aboriginal Living Skills School:* http://www.codylundin.com/

Made in the USA
Lexington, KY
06 December 2014